I'm Here

*Compassionate Communication
in Patient Care*

I'm Here

*Compassionate Communication
in Patient Care*

Marcus Engel

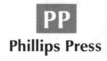

Phillips Press

Phillips Press
10961 Willow Ridge Loop
Orlando, FL 32825
407-913-0696
www.marcusengel.com

Printed in the United States of America
ISBN: 978-09720000-2-4

DEDICATION

For Barb DeWalle, R.N. and to the
memory of Mark DeWalle.
More than just a character in these books,
you saved my life,
literally and figuratively, many times.
I will always be honored to be your other Marc.

ACKNOWLEDGEMENTS

As always, this book would not be possible without the help of Marvelyne. Somewhere in the editing of *After This...* I fell in love with the most beautiful person I've ever known. It is a joy and a privilege to write with you, work with you and wake up with you every day, Mrs. Engel!

The following health care professionals offered their expertise in the writing of *I'm Here.*

Hilary Warren, M.D. Love ya, Hil... ever since our days in New Hall when I'd make you write my English reports while I drank cheap scotch, you have always been someone I can rely on. Thank you...

Timothy Jones, M.D. For putting me back together again and doing so in a way that gave me so much positive fodder for this career I've chosen in health care. Not everyone has a relationship with their physician where he/she would show up for the patient's wedding. Thank you for caring about me as a person, not just your patient.

Elaine Slater, R.N. Not only a character in my first two books, but someone who has cared for me since day one – literally.

To my parents, Phil and Nancy Engel, who proved you don't have to have R.N. or M.D. behind your name to provide loving, compassionate care.

Thanks also go to Beth Demoranville, R.N., Donna Wright, R.N. et aul from Creative Health Care Management, Kim Santos, R.N., Amanda Ransom, N.P., Dr. Albert Hall and staff, Richard Clark, P.A. and staff, Dr. Axel Castro and staff, Nicole Taylor, R.N. and last but not least, to you, faithful reader. I hope that within these pages, you'll find inspiration to encourage your care of patients and to continue the compassion shown to me during my recovery.

CONTENTS

FOREWORD

I am a child of the 80's. Those of us who were conceived while "All in the Family" was still on the tube are the first generation to grow up with instant everything. What is instant everything? Well, think of the good old days – I mean the REAL good old days like pre-1960. This is pretty tough for me since, well, I wasn't born until 1975. When I watch shows from the 50's or 60's, there is one thing that stands out: life just took forever!

Wanna bake cookies? Get the ingredients, sift the flour, wait for the butter to soften, yada yada yada. Making cookies from scratch nowadays is almost unthinkable. And why home make anything when everything can be purchased easier, cheaper and faster?

Around 1960 or so, the modern age came into being. Actually, most historians consider the modern age to have started sometime in the 50's. Why do I differ? Simple: The Rolling Stones. Ah yes, Mick Jagger, Keith Richards – those guys who've looked like corpses for the few decades leading up to their demise (at the writing of this sentence, they're not dead yet, but c'mon... we've all been expecting them to croak any minute since about 1988.)

More specifically than the band, I'm referring to the Stones' song, "Mother's Little Helper" the Stones first recorded in the 60's, hence my summation when the modern era began. Unscientific? Abso-freaking-lutely! I never claimed to be a historian!

Anyway, take "Mother's Little Helper." A song about drugs, basically. The mother in the song is worn out from the rigors of domestic life: cooking for her husband, taking care of unappreciative children, everything June Cleaver probably bitched about after penning "Dear Diary."

To combat the trials and tribulations of domesticity, "Mother" takes a little yellow pill, only to find she needs more and more and more. Who'd have thunk the Stones would have written the first anti-drug song? Go figure.

So, the vision of "Mother" helped usher in the modern era or, as I prefer to call it, the age of instant everything. Since the beginning of time, people have worked toward one common goal: make life easier. Inventions and discoveries helped push modernization along: fire, metal, the wheel, the printing press, Velcro shoes, automatic transmissions, the Slinky, you get it. Circa 1960 these inventions and modern marvels started to become so commonplace that each day pushed us one step closer to a life of ease.

About the time I can start consciously remembering things, Ronald Reagan was being sworn into office. Not only did Reagan's era scare the crap out of kids everywhere with thoughts of the Ruskies nuking us until we glowed a sickly green, but it also gave society the first true look at instant everything: video games, computers, microwaves, remote controls, VCRs, cable TV, ice makers, frozen burritos. If it's helped make us lazy, it's probably rooted in the 60's, but perfected in the 80's.

Why do I tell you all this? Partially an explanation, partially an excuse.

The age of instant everything coincided with the age of Marcus (that's me, by the way). I mean, I barely remember having to cross the room to slide the channel selector on the cable box. I remember getting our first microwave, but I sure don't remember life before it. Heating up leftovers in the oven? Are you kidding? How long did that take? 10, maybe 20 minutes? Who has time for that? There's Frogger to be played!

Even though I've been going on and on about this era of instant everything, I've failed to actually get to the freaking point already! Chalk that up to the Engel gift of gab. But, I digress once again. Stop me next time, okay?

So, instant everything. Those of us who grew up in the 80's, and every generation since, have never had to wait... on anything! This adds up to instant gratification, impatience and simply having short attention spans.

Here, I lead you into the reading of this book with a short story. Why short? Because you probably have a short attention span, too. And, if you want the long version, you'll read *After This... An Inspirational Journey for All the Wrong Reasons,* my 300 plus page autobiography. However, since you're holding this book for a purpose and you'll need a little background, I'll keep it brief. Here goes...

Your humble writer is me, Marcus Phillip Engel. Born in St. Louis, Missouri, I was raised in the suburbs for my first 10 years (that's where I learned to play Pong, got our microwave and typed on my first computer.) When I started the 4th grade, our family moved to a rural farming community 75 miles west of St. Louis. Growing up in High Hill, Missouri, I was your average red blooded American kid: little league, varsity football, high school band, choir, part time job at a Texaco service station... I even served on a few committees in my local church.

Three months after tossing my mortarboard with my graduating class of 1993 at Montgomery County R-II High School, the next phase of life began: college.

My freshman year at Missouri State University started with a bittersweet taste in my mouth. I'd loved high school and my teenage life and I hated to bid it farewell. Yet, this whole college thing was pretty exciting (not to mention there were tons of hot chicks!)

Three hours from my hometown, MSU was a perfect location for me to cut my teeth on life… but then, life cut its teeth on me.

Six weeks into my freshman year at Missouri State, I came home for a weekend with friends and family. Friday night high school homecoming football game, visiting with my parents, seeing my old teachers – I loved being back in that environment and showing that I was now a college man!

The weekend holiday also included a trip into the city to watch the home opener of my favorite hockey team, the St. Louis Blues. That game marked my last moments of normalcy… and the events after the final horn sounded are what led to this book currently resting in your hands. Those events aren't pretty – be prepared.

Following the game, we all piled into my friend's white Toyota Corolla. We pulled out of the parking lot, headed for home and maybe, just maybe, a stop at White Castle along the way.

The route was easy, Mackland Avenue to the south, Man-chester Road west, then Hampton Avenue south. We'd end up on the highway and, within 20 minutes, we'd be tucked into a corner table, chowing greasy cheeseburgers and chicken rings (yes, I said chicken rings, not chicken wings. If you're unacquainted with the best cuisine a half a buck can buy, stop into a White Castle and experience something special!).

A short distance down Hampton Avenue, we stopped for a red light. From my shotgun position, I glanced out my right window as soon as the light turned green. Headlights, a white car, the sound of crushing metal... then blackness and pain.

"Blackness and pain?" Those two words cannot begin to describe the intensity of these two perceptions. Blackness was a subterranean, haunted house, void of even the slightest tinge of color. No light, no shadows, no nothing. Thick as coagulated ink, darkness so powerful I could taste it. And pain? Christ Jesus, the pain.

The English language does not have a single word to illustrate the physical sensation from that scenario in the street. Picture the power of a car crusher. One of those hydraulic jobs that can mash a four door sedan into a condensed hunk of steel the size of a suitcase. Grinding Detroit metal, smashing together, side to side, back to front, flattening a Ford Taurus down to the size of an Igloo cooler. That was my face, my head, my body. But instead of the slow, deliberate motion of the crusher, think instantaneous. In the time it took you to flip the last page – just that quick. In the blink of an eye. Life, as you know it, is over. Welcome to my world.

In a heartbeat, I was blind. Blind AND living through one of the worst cases of facial trauma imaginable.

This is where the story for you begins. Please, step into my room in Barnes Hospital. Past the heavy wooden door. Through the extra wide threshold. Past the utilitarian bathroom and over to my bedside.

What do you see? Does that body look human? Maybe. Arms, legs, torso, hands, toes – all that seems to belong to a person. Scraped and black and blue and bloody, but certainly still human.

Then, let your eyes fall on the face. Humanistic – but not quite human. The proportions are all wrong. The forehead is swollen like a grotesque water balloon. The eyes are sewn shut with thick, black thread. The tubes that run into his (its'?) mouth make ghastly sucking sounds. Dried and fresh blood are everywhere, from the incision down the right cheek, to the jagged laceration across the jaw, to the scraped and oozing road rash that peeks out from the figure's sides and rear. Just a few teeth fragments can be seen through the thick, gorilla-like lips. Hear the hissing of the nearby tank as oxygen is pumped into the body's throat through a trach. Across it's lap lies a yellow legal tablet, complete with horrific scratches and jagged writing; the creature's only means of communication due to the trach.

That, is me. Me as an 18 year old kid, blind, suffering, hurting in ways no one should feel. And that horribly messed up kid hasn't yet been told all the details of the night he was brought in. Soon, though, thanks to the legal pad and pencil supplied by his Aunt Elaine, Marcus will get the news: this wreck, this damage, this darkness was all preventable. This absolute bludgeoning of his (my) body is the result of one person's action: the choice to drive drunk.

You may jump to the conclusion that Marcus and his friends, being teenagers out late at night, were knocking back a few cold ones. Negative. Instead, Marcus and his friends were the innocent party, ploughed down by an intoxicated driver. The knowledge of this fact fills the patient with an anger so tangible it's felt by everyone in the room, including you, the health care professional.

You get to observe the care Marcus now receives. You get to step into the shoes, the scrubs and the mind of his caregivers: his doctors, nurses, therapists, even the house-keeping and dietary staff. Or, you have the option to simply observe from afar. The choice is yours, but please notice the little bits of human interaction. These tiny glances, words, physical touches and conversations have the power to heal… and the power to hurt.

If you've read *The Other End Of The Stethoscope: 33 Insights For Excellent Patient Care*, you may remember some of these same situations. Chapter 1 is even exactly the same as Chapter 1 in "Stethoscope." Am I too lazy to write a totally new chapter? Hardly. The reason it's a re-run is because it's important. It is, simply put, the most comforting, compassionate, caring tip I hope you will take away from this book.

And in this age of instant everything, these chapters (dare I say… insights?) are kept short. My goal is not to waste your time dragging out a long-winded literary master-piece. Rather, I hope you'll pick up this book on your coffee break, smoke break or even when you step into the john. If you flip through a chapter or two, it should only take a few minutes… and I hope you'll absorb that info and take it with you into the care of your patients.

For our purposes now, we're going to leave the current day. Let us revert in time. To watch, to observe, to question and to learn. You will see health care professionals interact with that version of me. Some of these professionals epitomize what it means to care. Some are just selfish assholes who see this battered kid as nothing more than another load to their day. By the way, the names in this book of all the principal characters are real, and have my undying gratitude. Other names have been changed to protect the guilty.

But come in, pull up one of those uncomfortable chairs by my bedside and watch for a while. Hopefully, you'll learn some things.

MPE
February 2010
Orlando, FL

CHAPTER 1

Two Little Words

I keep hearing sounds: a siren, the clamor of EMS workers, the click of a stretcher as the wheels fall into place. Breaking glass, a woman screaming, the CB radio squawking in the ambulance. I can't put these sounds in order.

I can't listen to them.

I can't pay attention to them.

They just happen.

And they keep happening.

A woman shouts my name and orders me to lay still.

The 'whoosh' of automatic doors.

The taste of blood.

A warm blanket.

Pebbles of concrete under my hand.

And pain. God help me, the pain.

I was blind – immediately, totally, permanently; though no one would say for sure until the doctors had time to do some exploratory surgery. But, I knew. Deep down, I knew.

Now, here in the emergency room, white hot pain and utter confusion were my guides on the road to hell. Hands ravaged me. Hands everywhere. Cutting off my clothes, re-positioning my body, grabbing my arms and shoving needles into my flesh.

Gallons of morphine are pushed into an IV, it doesn't stop the pain, but it DOES get me so messed up on narcotics that I don't pay as much attention. The ability to think is completely shot. Memories don't hang around for more than a few seconds – then they're gone.

Exhaustion finally takes over and I fall into uncomfortable sleep. Even when I'm asleep, I hurt. God, the pain!

I awake with a mental crash landing. As soon as I grasp "this." This horror. This blackness. This rape of every square inch of my body. I'm bludgeoned into seeing white flashes of light. Not truly visual images, but the mental flashbulbs that explode with sudden pain. And they never stop. Paparazzi flashbulb explosions of pain. One after another. Pain is all I know. I surrender to it.

"Marcus? Can you hear me?" asks a female voice.

I dip my chin. A searing jolt slices my head back into place. I gasp. As I do, the sucking sound of inhalation comes from my throat. My throat? Not my mouth?

The owner of the voice slips her fingers into my right hand. With her other hand, she lightly traces two fingers up my forearm.

"Marcus, you're in Barnes Hospital. You were in a car accident," comes the soft voice again, "Just rest now."

I obey. Back into sleep, back to the haunted terrors of hallucination.

Maybe minutes, maybe hours later, I slam back into consciousness. I find the familiar hand from before.

Everything below the neck aches with a dull pain, and everything above burns like dipping my head into a blast furnace. Fear and hurt take over. My breathing kick starts to the rate of a sprinter.

Again, those same questions come from the girl.

"Marcus? Can you hear me?"

I'll be damned if I nod again and topple that boulder of pain. Instead, I squeeze the hand. She seems to understand. "Marcus, my name is Jennifer. You're in Barnes Hospital. You were in a car accident," Without thinking, I squeeze the hand again, just to show her I'm getting it.

She pauses. She gives my hand a soft squeeze. Then, the most comforting words of all, "I'm here."

I'm here. I don't even know where "here" is, other than some anonymous name like "Barnes Hospital." But I know I'm not alone. I'm hurt, I'm helpless and I'm scared. I cannot be alone. I cannot be alone. And she's here. This Jennifer girl with her soft hand and quiet voice. She's here.

Jennifer doesn't say her title, doesn't give her background nor her credentials, just bare bones information. Nothing else is necessary; and she knows it. All I need to know is that in this world of black – this ocean of pain, I am not alone.

⟨⎯⎯⟩

"I'm here." Those two little words are a verbal embrace, a warm, safe place of protection for your patient. Patients relinquish all independence, all pride and all needs to you. Those words, "I'm here," give an anchor of security and reassurance. No one wants to be alone, especially in an unfamiliar place

and with strange things happening. No one wants to be in a hospital, out of their usual element of safety and familiarity. Throw in the pain and fear of whatever their ailment entails and sometimes reassurance is what your patient needs most.

"I'm here" also secures your role as the caregiver. Let's just face it; the patient/caregiver relationship is similar to a child and parent. While the caregiver is on duty, they become the parent. The patient longs for the comfort that all children desire; knowledge that their parent is nearby and watching over them.

Those two simple little words can offer more hope and security than anything else you can say or do. As you leave one patient to attend another, use those two little words to reassure your patient that he/she is safe, secure and that all is well. Try it. You'll see your patient's comfort level raise and raise.

CHAPTER 2

"He's Doing Good"

I can barely comprehend anything around me. Everything, I mean EVERYTHING screams out in pain. My head feels like someone is crushing it in a vice grip. My face is so swollen it feels as though I'm suffocating. My ear, my arms, my chest, my back, my legs – every square inch of my body feels like I took a beating with a lead pipe. With each person who enters the room, there is the chance of more pain. If a question is asked of me, the best I can do is nod or shake my head. Either of these motions sets off the single worst sensation I've ever experienced; hearing AND feeling fluid inside my skull. This isn't like inner ear fluid, but it sounds like it's coming from the back of my head. *Is my brain swimming in there? If I tilt my head, will I become brain dead?*

I'm scared. The doctors say I'll never see again, that my face has been crushed, that I'm looking forward to a few hundred hours of surgery. I mourn these facts, but there's no time for emotions. Plus, I'm empty. There's no energy for feelings, just enough energy to try to keep me from hurting. And the best way to keep from hurting is to lay still. Still like a dead man. Still like an immovable boulder. Still like night in the desert. I will not move. I won't flinch, won't twitch, will not do anything but breathe. And those breaths will come shallow and light. If I can remain still, maybe the pain will subside… maybe, just a little.

A nurse enters the room. She glances at me, sees that I'm not moving. She turns to my parents and whispers, "I just need to check his vitals."

Everything is automated: the blood pressure cuff on my arm, the oximeter on my finger, my IV drugs, the O_2 tank that pumps life-giving air into my lungs. While I'm fully conscious, with all these machines and tubes and drugs, it still adds up to one thing: life support.

The nurse comes around my bed. She whispers her presence. I do not move. She nudges the bed with her hip as she reaches above me to check the flow of the IV bag. There's a slight twinge of fear that's over before it starts – just enough to scare me, not enough to hurt me. But fear of the pain keeps me on edge.

The nurse finishes her tasks. She grabs the chart from the end of my bed and begins to write.

"His blood pressure, oxygen, heart rate and breathing are all holding steady. He's doing good, Mr. and Mrs. Engel."

Doing good? I'd done nothing "good" since coming under her care. My life was still precariously balanced somewhere between "death" and "close to death."

Yet, my vitals were all strong. This nurse was certain of that. My parents didn't have much to hold onto at that moment, but hearing that I was doing good – even if I wasn't doing anything different – gave them some hope and comfort that I wasn't going to die.

If your patient isn't showing any improvement, but is holding steady, consider that something good. And communicating that stability to the patient and his/her family might be the only good news they get. Whatever opportunity you have to reassure the patient and his/her family, do it. Hope springs eternal.

CHAPTER 3

"You're In The Best Place!"

"Hi, Marcus… I'm Barb, your new nurse," comes a female voice from the side of my bed. "Welcome to the 7400 floor." The voice is strong and confident, speaking to me directly.

"And we're here, too, Brother," says my dad, off to the side and a short distance away.

I try to respond, but the yawning sound comes from my throat. No words, thanks to the trach. Instead of talking, I dip my head in a barely perceptible nod.

"As soon as I get all these tubes hooked up, your folks can come over here and hold your hand, okay, Marcus?"

I nod again. The sloshing and rolling of fluid is still present, but to a much lesser degree.

"You had a big operation, Marcus – nearly 24 hours. This is the post surgical unit you're on now and we get to take care of you from now on!" Barb sounds genuinely pleased.

Gets to take care of me? Well, good to know she doesn't think it's a chore.

Barb shuffles around my bed, marking things on the chart, arranging the IV bag to drip properly, seeing what medications my surgeon, Dr. Jones, has ordered.

"Have you ever been in the hospital, Marcus?" I nod and make a writing motion with my hand.

"He wants his tablet," says Mom. She hands the tablet to Barb who hands it to me.

"*Yes, twice,*" I scrawl, mute from the trach.

"For what?" Barb asks. She pauses, focusing on our communication.

"*Hernias from football,*" I write.

"Where did you have those surgeries?"

I can hear the interest written across her face.

Barb is seeing that, as messed up as I am, my brain was not damaged in the wreck.

I scrawl out the name of the hospital where, a year ago, I'd undergone an operation for a hernia repair.

"Well, I've gotta tell ya, Marc, you're in for a treat! You're in Barnes Hospital now… and Barnes is the best hospital around! We're always ranked as one of the top 10 hospitals in the whole country!"

Barb's enthusiasm is nothing short of contagious. Through the pain, the grogginess, the morphine, the knowledge… Barb's energy shines through!

"And ya know what's even better than that, Marcus? This floor you're on now is 7400… and we are absolutely, positively the best floor in the whole hospital! You just wait and see!"

I won't bother to correct her about "seeing" anything, I'm just happy she's talking to me like a real person.

"*Good,*" I write out, feeling fatigue envelop me.

25

"Just a couple more little things I have to do here, Marc. Then I'll give you some morphine and we'll let you sleep, okay?" Barb arranges items on my new bedside table. I nod. There's nothing fun about this. I hurt like holy hell, I can't see, I can barely move… but I know I'm in a good place and I have someone who seems like she's going to take good care of me.

Any opportunity you get, compliment your employer. How often do you hear people complain about their boss, their manager, their co-workers, or their work environment? Probably every day. This is not a great way to get ahead anywhere – but is completely unacceptable in a health care institution. Caregivers have the opportunity to help patients feel their care will be exceptional!

First and foremost, reassure your patient that he/she is in a competent, capable place. Second, it's great to hear how caregivers love their employer.

A happy, satisfied worker is more likely to be fully engaged with all aspects of their work environment. This means they're less likely to make mistakes and MORE likely to help create a self-fulfilling prophecy about the patient's care.

Nearly every health care institution can find some kind of award, recognition or ranking that says they're a quality place to be treated. So be proud! Sharing this info can help reassure the patient that he/she is in good hands!

CHAPTER 4

"We Have The Best Staff – Anywhere!"

B arb is again at my bedside. I've been resting… sort of. Sleep may be present, but it's hard to differentiate between it and hallucinations.

"Hey Marc," she says quietly, cautiously checking to see if I'm conscious. I lift a hand to show her I comprehend.

"My shift is over in 30 minutes. I just wanted to be sure you're comfortable before I go…"

I nod. I just want to sleep.

"Okay, I'll tell your next nurse you've been trying to sleep. By the way, his name is Rick and you're going to love him!"

I nod, a little more intrigued. So far, all of my nurses have been female. It'll be interesting to have another guy taking care of me.

"Rick is just awesome!" Barb exclaims quietly. "We call him the king of the ICU! He's really, really good at what he does. You'll probably also meet Betty this afternoon, I think her shift starts at 3. Betty is an LPN and she's been on this floor for almost 20 years… even longer than me!" I nod my comprehension. If Barb likes them, I probably will, too!

"Yeah, Betty has gotten all kinds of awards from the hospital and is always being nominated by her co-workers. You'll also meet Stephanie. She's a new nurse, but all her patients seem to love her!"

⟡

Have you ever gotten a compliment through the grapevine? We're all accustomed to receiving obligatory accolades , but when we receive a compliment that wasn't spoken directly to us, it carries more weight. Barb's compliments for Rick, Betty and Stephanie showed how much she cares about them... AND how much she cares about me!

Every opportunity you have, compliment your co-workers to your patient. Even if they're not your favorite person, it helps your patient. Patients want to know they're under the care of competent, quality individuals. And they're also placing a lot of trust in each and every caregiver. If one caregiver gives props to the next on duty, the patient is reassured that their care will be seamless.

I want to know that, if I had a problem while Barb was on duty, my next nurse will be kept abreast of the situation. We talk more to people we like, less to those we don't. Patients want to know their caregivers are talking, insuring a flawless transfer.

CHAPTER 5

It Rolls Downhill

I wake from a nightmare. Gasping sounds come from my neck. The dream, I realize, was just that, a dream. But the intensity is physically resonating within my skull. I nod, shifting my head to figure out if I'm truly awake. The sickening slosh of fluid in the rear of my skull sounds a ghastly alarm. I halt all movement, trying to hear if the breathing from my trach is regular. *Hiss, suck, hiss, suck.* This audio inhalation and exhalation, creepy as it is, means everything is okay. My trach is open. Oxygen freely flows to my lungs. I will not suffocate... at least, not right now.

I relax. *Breathing, check. Nightmare over, check. Understand the reality of this hell I'm in, check...sorta.* That nightmare, the raw, gripping fear that I was suffocating, the terror of being unable to move the weight from my chest – it's just still so real. Definitely one of the most vivid nightmares since childhood. *What brought this on? The reality of my life? The drugs? The drugs – definitely the drugs.*

"No more of that stuff," I think, remembering the drug inserted in my IV a few hours before. Some pleasant-sounding name: halcion, serenity, euphoria, something that sounded nice. *Lying drugs. If this nightmare is any indication of how bad this stuff jacks up my brain, I'm done with it.*

I shift slightly in the bed. As I move, there's 'something' between my legs. I push a slow hand under the sheet, the blanket, my gown; exploring. My fingertips touch the flesh of my thigh. I trace my fingers towards my crotch, afraid of what this foreign "stuff" is in my bed. An inch further, a finger dips into a thick 'something.' Not warm, not cold, it's the consistency of lumpy mud. *Mud? How did I get mud in my bed?*

I push my index and middle fingers down further. *Blood? No, too thick. Did I piss the bed? Too thick for that, too.* I pull my hand back, feeling the stickiness between my thumb, index and middle fingers. A clump falls off and I feel the weight stick to my gown. Slowly, I pull my fingers toward my nose. As always, there is no smell. Even the most pungent, wretched odor can't penetrate the swelling and damage to my olfactory system. My sense of smell is simply gone… right along with my sight. I wipe my fingers on my gown and push a hand to the edge of the bed. There, on the rail, the nurse call button is secured with bandage tape. I press it and wait.

A few minutes later, a nurse tech scurries in.

"What's that on your gown, Marcus?" she asks. I shrug my shoulders and shake my head. Then… she gasps.

My heart rate skyrockets.

What's wrong? What is this stuff?

"Be right back," she says over her shoulder, footsteps walking quickly out of the room. I take another breath, scared. She returns a few moments later, along with another set of footsteps.

"Hey, buddy, it's Barb," the second voice says. *Yes! Barb is here! She'll solve the mystery of the mud!*

"Can you get me a couple warm wet rags?" Barb asks the nervous tech.

She steps to the bedside. ""You ready for a quick sponge bath, buddy?" *Sponge bath? For what?*

Barb gently lifts my wrist. The warm water and wash-cloth give some pleasant sensations in this world of pain. Down my fingertips, across the knuckles, down my palm slides the wash cloth. Once Barb is finished cleaning my hand, I make a writing motion. Barb doesn't hand the tablet over immediately, so I snap my fingers and fane writing more urgently.

"Give me just a minute, Marcus. I've gotta get you cleaned a little before I can get your tablet."

Cleaned?

"It's okay, I've got this," Barb says to the nurse tech.

"Are you sure?" The tech sounds barely old enough to drive, much less to take care of patients.

"Sure, this is no big deal... right Marcus?"

I shrug again. I don't even know what "this" is. But, I trust Barb. If she says it's no big deal, then it isn't. "No big deal at all," she says again, drying my hand with another towel. I wait for her to finish this task.

"Here ya go," she says, handing over my tablet.

"What is that?" I write. She repeats each word as it's completed.

"Well, Marcus, I think you had an accident."

An accident?

I'm not sure Barb understands the question, so I push my fingers below my robe, back to the coagulated mess.

31

Again, my fingers come away with the substance all around. Again, she takes my hand and rubs a damp (and now cool) washrag around each digit. Even through my nerve damaged and swollen face, the confusion shows through. I turn my palm up in a gesture to say, *"What is this?"*

"Ohhh," Barb says, drawing out the "O" in a sound of realization. She gets it; she understands that I do NOT understand.

"Marcus, I think you had an accident. Do you remember going to the bathroom?"

The bathroom? I can't get out of bed without four people lifting me from the bed, sling-like, in a sheet pulled taut. How could I have gotten up by myself and gone to the bathroom?

Then, it hits me. *Bathroom? Bathroom! This mess between my legs – this sticky, cooling mess, it's my own shit.* I realize, horrified, I've been dipping my fingers into my own waste! For the first time since I was a toddler, I've crapped the bed. *But, how? The mess between my legs wasn't warm. That doesn't make sense, does it?.... Unless I've been lying in it so long it's gotten cold.* The realization falls on me like a boulder from sky high. I just shit the bed, I just shit the bed. I want to cry, I want to vomit, I want to weep in the arms of my favorite nurse for making such a horrible, filthy mess of her night. And yet? I don't remember anything – not one little bit. I've laid in my own mess for, what? Hours? I'm beyond disgusting, I think silently, ready to weep. I'm sick with shame. I grab the pencil as my body racks with silent sobs.

"I'm so so sorry," I write, over and over again. I loathe my helplessness, am afraid of not remembering anything

and hate, HATE that Barb has to wipe me like I'm a baby in diapers.

"Marcus," Barb says, a bit of surprise and dismay in her voice. "It's okay, it's all okay. This is an easy fix. I'll get you cleaned up and help you get back to bed so you can sleep. I promise this isn't a big deal..."

Barb has 20 plus years of nursing experience. The nurse tech? Maybe 20 days. Yet, who cleaned me up? Who took on the most despised job of a health care professional? Barb could have easily handed down the task to the lowest man on the totem pole-but she didn't. Instead, she took on the responsibility, shouldered the task and gave the nurse tech the ability to walk away.

More importantly, Barb gave me some comfort and security to have this task performed by her, not a stranger. Did Barb do this because of our relationship? Maybe, but either way, it emphasized a couple great points for patient care.

First, she took into account my utter horror and embarrassment at having crapped the bed. Second, even though Barb had superiority, she gave the nurse tech a pass on a not-so-coveted job.

In health care, like in so many other professions, the shit rolls downhill (no pun intended). Sad as it is, many times those in superior positions pass the buck to their subordinates. This willingness to sink to the level of doing an underling's job showed the truest compassion for the patient.

CHAPTER 6

"You Have To Do What Is Right For You"

"Hey, Marcus," Dr. Jones says, giving the door a quick courtesy knock as he strides into the room.

"*Hi*," I write. He'd get no more from me, unless we were going to discuss what would happen from here. For now? I'm just aggravated. Why? Because Dr. Jones, this plastic surgeon standing next to me, had prescribed two drugs that'd become the bane of my existence: a stool softener and the sleeping drug that worked so well I wasn't even conscious when the stool softener kicked in. After Barb helped me get clean, I'd written, *"I'm not taking those drugs anymore."* Barb had protested.

"Marcus, with all the surgery you're having, you really need to take the stool softener. Anesthesia makes your intestines clog up and you'll be constipated."

I'd turned my thumb upside down. It was final. Well, to me it was. Barb tried a few different angles. First, it was my own health. Then it was how she'd be proud of me if I took the stool softener. No dice, still not gonna do it. Thirdly and finally, she'd said, "Dr. Jones prescribed you these medications and I'm sure he wants you to take them."

"I'll take it up with him," I'd written. With that final scrawl, the conversation was over.

Now, Dr. Jones stands next to my bed. "Was there a problem with your medication, Marcus?" he asks, sounding truly concerned.

"I shit the bed and didn't know it. I'm not taking those drugs anymore," I write.

Dr. Jones sighs. "Well, you've got to do what's right for you, Marcus. I'd like you to continue to take the stool softener to keep your bowels working properly. The other drug is just to help you sleep."

"I don't care. That stuff is horrible."

"Okay, Marcus – it's your choice. Again, you have to do what is right for you."

⟵⟶

No matter your role as a health care professional, your goal has to be to help your patient. If you are a physician and the patient makes a conscious choice not to heed your advice, so be it; you are there to help them get better. If they do not, the burden is on them. If you're a nurse, tech, etc., your goal has to be, again, to help the patient. Barb encouraged me to keep taking the medications. In her heart, she was watching out for me – not just trying to follow doctor's orders.

Be sure that your job isn't ONLY being done to fulfill a physician's orders – but that you're trying to help the patient. If your patient refuses to help him/herself, being Zen about their care is the best angle: Mr./Ms. Patient, you must do what's right for you.

CHAPTER 7

"Nasty Wound"

My butt hurts – severely. The skin on each cheek is simply gone. Scraped off by the pavement, my thighs, over my rear and onto my back is a condition called, "Road Rash." Patches the size of a hand are red, angry wounds oozing fluid. Unable to move, bedsores have erupted on top of the road rash. Every couple hours large men turn me from side to side. Even the slightest jostling of my robe sends avalanches of pain throughout my body, so every time these orderlies show up to do their work, I pray for death. *Pain this intense cannot even exist*, I tell myself, as volcanic explosions batter my head, inside out.

Here, lying on my side, the road rash and bed sores are supposed to be exposed to the outside air. This means my bare ass is on display for the entire world to see. Plus, nurses have to treat these injuries. Polysporin, alcohol, dressings – their arsenal is extensive. And I'm embarrassed. And in pain. And I hate, HATE this process.

"I know this isn't real comfy, Marcus, but you've got some really nasty wounds and they have to be treated. I'll be done in just a few minutes, okay?" I nod a reply. I hold my breath and scrunch up my face, just trying to get through it.

The fiery alcohol burning across my "nasty wounds" makes me howl in pain… at least, I would howl if I could make the slightest vocal inflection, which I cannot. The meager amounts of breath I can draw in this position scare me – I need to breathe. And this nurse still messes with my butt – not since infancy has someone had to powder my butt and rub cream on my crotch. I am simply humiliated at the need to take care of me like I'm a baby.

And all the while I keep thinking about this "nasty wound."

Black mold is nasty. Cheap German skin flicks are nasty. Severe halitosis is nasty.

I don't want anything nasty to be associated with my body. Even though she's right – the wound IS nasty; her comment makes me feel responsibility for just how gross this is.

Instead of commenting on how nasty, disgusting, awful, etc. an incision site or wound is, find something to compliment about the area. Highlight the positive, don't comment on the negative. Try out these: "The wound looks like it's healing nicely" or "This incision site looks healthy" or "There's no infection here, so we'll just keep treating it to prevent anything bad from happening." Again, magnify the positive, diminish the negatives. And if the wound truly is nasty? Keep the color commentary to yourself.

CHAPTER 8

"Can I have a look at this?"

Tomorrow is gonna suck. After another night of what is sure to be a time of gut wrenching anxiety and insomnia, I'll be wheeled out of this room, down the hall, into the elevator, down another hall and into pre-op. The requisite IV's will be started, marks made upon my body, drugs shot into my veins, sleepy euphoria will take over and Dr. Jones (and half a dozen other surgeons) will begin some new procedures.

What will these be? I dunno. I don't want to think about it. I'm sick to death of surgery, sick to death of being in the recovery room, my mouth aching for water, my head feeling as though it's just been inflated to bursting. I hate this… and yet? There's no choice. If I ever want to get out of this place, if I ever want to swallow a lungful of air outside this sterile hospital, I have to put one foot in front of the other and allow the surgeons to do what they need to do. I have to do this, but it doesn't change my hatred.

Dr. Jones has secured his role as my primary plastic surgeon. The first couple of times he's worked on me, I was so doped up and out of my head with pain that a first impression was impossible… or simply forgotten. Now? He's fine. I take comfort in the fact he's not only a plastic surgeon, but he's also an ear, nose and throat surgeon. And with ears, nose and throat as damaged as mine, having a switch hitter of a surgeon is exactly what I need.

"Marcus, it's Dr. Jones," he says, rousing me from a fitful nap. I half nod, half shrug to show I understand.

"Tomorrow morning Dr. Neely and I are going to reconstruct your ear canal. We're also going to bridge your left facial nerve." I nod again, more out of politeness than anything.

"I'm going to touch your arm, Marcus," Dr. Jones says. I'm pleased he remembers that I can't see his hands moving toward me. Any unannounced touch is shocking, complete with a gasp and recoil.

Dr. Jones, slowly, gingerly lifts the short sleeve of my gown. He rolls it and tucks it high on my arm like a pack of ciggies rolled up in the white T-shirt of a 1950's greaser. Keeping one hand on my wrist, he moves a single finger to my bicep. In a long, straight line, he moves his finger from my armpit to elbow.

"We'll take a nerve from right here, Marcus." He gently taps the area he has just traced. "Over here under your left ear," he says, lifting his hands from my arm and gliding around the bed, "This is where we'll bridge that severed facial nerve." I sense, rather than feel, a fingertip under my earlobe. It moves down my jaw line and stops somewhere near the trach.

"When this nerve was severed, it paralyzed the left side of your face. The nerve from your bicep area will go in here and that should help you regain some sensation. Nerve regeneration takes a long, long time. If everything works as it

39

should, you may begin to have some feeling back in a few months." I shrug again. I don't really want to hear about this, I just want it to be over.

My parents ask questions. I zone out. Purposefully. Dr. Jones and Mom and Dad discuss tomorrow's surgery. I think about music, about high school, about the pillow under my head – anything that is NOT about surgery.

A Bruce Springsteen song plays on the stereo. There is chatter from nurses in the hallway. An announcement from the P.A.

"Does that sound okay with you, Marcus?" Dr. Jones asks. I snap back into the here and now. The right side of my face scrunches up in a look of questioning confusion.

"Your leg, do you mind if I have a look?" I nod and make a "Go ahead" gesture.

My leg? What's he want to see my leg for?

The sheet and blanket are slowly lifted from my left side. Cool air penetrates sweaty, unwashed skin on my thigh. "Hey! That's looking really good, big guy!" Dr. Jones' pleasure is genuine.

My leg? What does a plastic surgeon care about my leg?

"The last time I was in here, your legs were still hanging in traction. This fixator is a big piece of hardware, but it looks like Dr. Perry did a great job with this! We'll be sure the O.R. team is gentle with this tomorrow, okay, Marcus?" I nod and give a thumbs up.

⸺

Was Dr. Jones operating on my leg? Would anyone in the O.R. have anything to do with the external fixator on my lower half?

Did Dr. Jones have any reason, other than professional curiosity, for wanting to examine my orthopedic handiwork? No, no and no.

Yet? I was ecstatic that he did! Why? Dr. Jones made a conscious effort to look at me as a whole person. Even though he'd be doing nothing from the chest down, his interest in how my leg was healing made me feel as though I was an individual, not just tomorrow's surgical patient.

Patients never want to be seen as a procedure. If you see an old surgery scar, ask about it. Patients always want to know they are being considered holistically, not just as parts and procedures.

CHAPTER 9

State Your Title,
Not Just Your Task

"Hello, Engel family," says a new voice. Male, confident, gentle.

"I'm Gene Deune. I'll be assisting Dr. Jones tomorrow."

This Gene Deune character walks to my bed, shakes my right hand, and turns to my parents. He walks toward them, shakes their hands and sits down.

"I'd like to give you some information on what will be happening tomorrow," he says, focusing his attention on Mom and Dad. I'm too stoned on narcotics to pay much attention. Hell, I do not WANT to pay attention. I don't want to hear whatever he's going to say. I don't want to think about the pain, the incisions, the pre-op, the recovery room, the horror of it all. I force myself to zone. Back, back to the place where I detect the sensations I want to detect: the beep of my IV drip, the distant flush of a toilet down the hall, the DJ talking on the radio next to my bed. Anything, ANYTHING that is not Gene Deune's description of my tomorrow.

Yet, I'm not successful. From the end of my bed, snatches of conversation penetrate my forced solitude. Words like operation, bone graft, nose, plates travel from Gene Deune's mouth to my ears. Well, my ear, singular. My right ear is swollen and functioning. My left? So much pain, so many dressings, stitches, blood. No sound can enter the left side of my auditory system.

After a few more minutes, Gene Deune stands. "I'll see you tomorrow morning, Marcus," I dip my head in a nod. He exits.

I lift my hand and make a writing motion. Mom places my tablet and clipboard and pencil on my lap.

"*Who is he?*" I write.

"Gene Deune," my dad says, repeating information I already knew.

Duh, I got that much! I don't have enough energy to point out Dad's inept description.

"*Is he a doctor?*" I scrawl.

"I'm pretty sure he is," says my mom. "He was wearing scrubs and a white coat. I think he's one of Doc Jones' residents."

"*He should have said that,*" I print.

⟨⟩

After this meeting, Gene Deune would announce his presence. "Hey Marcus, Gene Deune from plastic surgery." He was, in fact, Dr. Jones' resident. Yet, he never identified himself as Dr. Gene Deune." On one hand, I appreciated his informality. He wasn't one enamored with his title. On the other hand, I didn't know what "resident" even meant. I could figure out the diff between doctor and nurse, but residency was something I didn't get. Are you a doctor? Not a doctor?

With so, so many people going in and out of my hospital room, and focusing only on voices, it became so important to know what each person's title was. Unless someone has a name tag, the average patient cannot distinguish between one person in scrubs and the next. Don't be afraid to re-introduce yourself and state your title. Many patients, like many people, would quickly admit, "I'm not good with names." This is why repeatedly telling the patient your name AND position is so important.

CHAPTER 10

Pillow Talk For
Private Parts

I have a new nurse. She seems nice enough. We're preparing for a big surgery. Lovely.

The drugs are really tearing up my mind. My short term memory is just shot. Tell me something, and you'll have to tell me again in just a few seconds. Just that quick. Plus, my ear is packed with some sort of substance. I picture it as a clay or gum, but truthfully, I don't know what it is. All I know is that I can't hear out of my left side. I'm totally blind, half deaf, and stoned. Drugs and disability are the rules of the game tonight. This nurse… Paula? I think her name is, said she'll be back in a few minutes. I lay and wait. When she returns, she pulls up a seat next to my bed.

"I'll be right here until they take you down to surgery, Marcus. That should be in just a couple hours." I nod. She's speaking loud, probably knowing I can't read lips, my hearing is half gone and maybe, just maybe, she's had to yell through the stoned mindsets of many a patient.

"Do you want me to tell you what will happen when they take you to pre-op, Marcus?" I nod again. Her voice is strong and sure. She definitely knows what she's talking about. I'm a little embarrassed that she's having to speak to me, an 18 year old guy, like we did to my hearing impaired late grandfather. Still, I want the information.

"The orderlies will take you to pre-op. There, a tech will probably shave the areas where the doctors will be operating. They'll probably also give you some nice drugs to relax before taking you into surgery. You'll still have your mom and dad with you, too. Then, they'll roll you into an operating room and you'll be fast asleep." I nod my comprehension.

"After surgery, you'll go to the recovery room where you'll start to wake up."

I sort out the bits I can comprehend. Pre-op, parents, shave, operating room, recovery room. She leans back in her chair, seemingly with a bit of renewed energy… and an extra bit of volume.

"The recovery room nurses will make sure everything is okay when you're waking up. You'll probably have an oxygen mask on, and you'll likely be full of morphine and other drugs. Oh, and you'll have a foley catheter, too."

Foley catheter? I furrow my brow, hoping she'll notice.

"Do you know what a foley catheter is, Marcus?"

I shake my head.

Her voice and demeanor soften. She leans close to my good ear. The volume has dropped and the conversation continues – but quietly.

"It's a tube that is in your penis. It carries urine from your bladder to a bag. Your bladder will take some time to wake up after surgery. The foley will keep your bladder working right until your body fully wakes up from surgery."

When you have to speak about a patient's private parts, or a procedure they may be embarrassed of, lower your voice. Lean close, speak clearly and quietly. Also, for patients who are NOT blind, be sure to face them (you never know how much you read lips until you're not able to see the person talking).

With all the HIPAA rules and regs about who can and cannot see your files and know your health history, the health care world seems to have forgotten one thing: oral communication. People can hear most everything you say to your patient. The other patients in the room, the staff, a variety of people who do not need to know your patient's business.

But, common sense should dictate that when you're talking to a patient about embarrassing things or their nether regions, keep your communication quiet. Pillow talk for private parts sounds like something you'd find on the magazine shelf at a truck stop, but try to keep it in mind for patients, too.

CHAPTER 11

Introduce Yourself,
No Matter Your Role

"We're going down to pre-op," says an unfamiliar male voice. Metal clanks around my bed as IV's and tubes and wires are prepped for transport.

"We're here, Brother," my dad says. He's far away. My world has now been reduced to whatever I can hear. And whatever is in my reach: the bed rails, my pillows, the end of the bed. My world is barely bigger than a casket. When people speak to me, it's almost always while they hold my hand. This lets me know they are close. Now, even though I can hear Dad, he is far, far away.

In reality, he's just out of reach. Just beyond the walls of my casket. I stretch out a hand toward him, but he doesn't take it. He's hanging back to let these anonymous men do their work. And their job is to get me from point A to point B.

Suddenly, I'm moving. I can feel the slightest hint of air wash over my hands and the right side (the non-dead) side of my face.

The bed stops. No one speaks. A bell dings. *An elevator?* The bed begins to roll. The bed bumps across the threshold into the elevator. My brain and body jolt. Fluid sloshes in the rear of my skull. I make a tight fist with my hands and hold my breath. The sound changes. Inside the elevator now. The tone of the bell again. The bed begins to roll out. The cool breeze flutters by. I want more of it. To drink in that cool air, to taste fresh oxygen. When the bed is still, it never even occurs to me to want fresh air. Now? With everything inside me, I long for the tiniest wisp of cold, clean air.

The bed stops. We seem to have arrived at our destination. *Pre-op?* The unknown men begin the reversal of their task. More clanking of tubes hitting metal. My parents whisper, "Thank you" as the men move along to their next task. Metal hooks slide overhead. "Let's give you a little privacy, Marc," my mom says. More metal scratches. The curtains around my bed don't block out the noise of anything, but if this privacy makes my parents feel better, let it be. Their hands come to me, holding and comforting.

No one speaks.

The metal hooks scrape again. Greetings are murmured between my parents and someone who has just entered my sanctum. "I'm going to get your blood pressure," says an unknown female voice. I hear the ripping of Velcro as the cuff is fixed around my right bicep. Six, seven, eight squeaky sounds of air as my arm is squeezed. I can feel the throbbing of the circulation. The release of the cuff, the pressure. The female voice says, "Thank you." Metal hooks scrape overhead.

Who the hell was that? I wonder. *A nurse? An anesthesiologist?* I truly have no idea, other than she was female and apparently took my blood pressure.

These interactions took less than 10 minutes. From the time the orderlies arrived, got me situated and transported to the pre-op area until the blood pressure taker did her job was far, far less time than it takes to watch a Thursday night sit-com.

There was no harm done. No one hurt me, insulted me, treated me like anything but a patient. Yet, the health care professionals missed some great opportunities. While their jobs weren't to be hand holders, no one likes to feel as though they are being bounced around by anonymous people.

Think of this… the orderlies could have easily said, "Marcus, my name is Ed and my partner here is Jeff. We're orderlies and we're going to transport you down to pre-op."

Why did the orderlies and the blood pressure girl not introduce themselves? Simply put, I think many health care professionals know their interactions with patients will be brief. They feel a formal introduction is unnecessary due to their role, or the time they'll be performing their task. Same thing with whoever took my BP in pre-op. I wasn't necessarily afraid of her, but she missed a chance to offer me a personal touch and some security.

Any time you interact with a patient, be sure to state your name and your role – no matter what that role is. A nurse on the hospital floor often establishes a relationship with his/her patient due to the time spent together. However, even if the health care pro's task only takes a few moments, one's name, title and task can leave a lasting impression.

CHAPTER 12

Taking Care Of Patients
Who Are Not Your Patients

"Any questions, Marcus?" Dr. Jones asks. I shake my head, ever so slightly, trying not to move. Yesterday was a 15 hour facial reconstruction, the second in as many weeks. Less than 20 days into this nightmare, the tragedy has softened a bit, but the trauma continues.

"Mr. and Mrs. Engel, do you have any questions?" He directs his question over the bed, across my body, to where my parents sit holding my hand and stroking my arm for comfort.

"I don't think so," they mumble.

"If you do have questions, just call my office. I'll be sure to swing up here and see what's up. But, I have a question for you two…"

Dr. Jones pauses, measuring his words. Mom and Dad sit silently, holding my hand.

"How are you guys doing?"

He pauses again, allowing them to answer in their own time. Empathy just exudes from his voice. Dr. Jones is a parent, too. He's watched Mom and Dad keep vigil at my bedside for weeks. He's seen their tears as I've been rolled into the operating room. He's heard despair in their voices as they've chatted with him privately.

"I think we're okay," my dad says. He doesn't sound okay. Mom is unable to answer. She takes a deep, choppy breath.

"You guys are here so much," Dr. Jones says, softening his voice further. "I know Marcus needs you around and I know you want to be by his side. But are you both getting enough sleep?"

Dad shrugs, but neither parent answers.

Dr. Jones continues. "I'm not your treating physician, but I can put you in touch with anyone Washington University and Barnes Hospital has on staff."

"Okay," Dad says, resigned. His answer is one of understanding, not acceptance. He seems… beaten up.

"If you guys need medications for sleep or anything else, there are doctors who specialize in helping families after a tragedy. There is also a really good counseling staff here at the hospital. Again, you have my number and just let me know if I can help put you in touch with anyone, okay?"

"Thank you," Mom and Dad whisper in unison. Both quiet, both exhausted, both grateful beyond words.

Every health care professional's primary goal is to take care of the patient. Sometimes, though, that means helping the family of the patient. Dr. Jones came to feel Mom and Dad's pain, not as a surgeon, but as a parent.

Even as wrecked as I was, I knew to the best of my 18 year old ability, that my parents were also hurting. I'll never be able to fully grasp the depths of their hell. Yet, I gained comfort knowing Dr. Jones and many, many other of my caregivers were also looking out for them.

Patients aren't stupid. They're not oblivious. They know that seeing them hurt is hard on their family members. If you can also help the family members, you are helping your patient.

Barb did this in her role as a nurse. Bringing my mom a cup of coffee, or just taking her into the hall to give her some support, those tiny little acts of care and support are often the only points of light in the day of the patient's family.

CHAPTER 13

"Any Questions?"

"I'll be taking a measure of skin from your waistline, Marcus," Dr. Jones says, pointing to an area just above my hip socket. "It'll be a fairly small piece; nothing like when we took the rib from your chest. We like to use skin from this area because there's generally not a lot of hair." He turns to my parents, giving us all the explanation.

"I'll then graft that portion of skin into your mouth. The fistula on your upper pallet can be closed twice. I'll first sew it shut like simply sewing a hole closed. Then, I'll cover the whole area with the skin graft, much like putting a patch on a pair of jeans. It should cover all the exposed bone in your oral cavity."

This will not be fun. Even if the piece of skin is small, there'll be an incision on my hip. And then anything inside my mouth tends to feel gigantic. Dr. Jones continues.

"Unfortunately, the oral cavity is very fragile. There's no place that's harder to graft skin to than the inside of the mouth. This surgery can succeed, but it'll require a lot of steps and really following my orders, okay, Marcus?" I nod. I'll do whatever he says.

"First off, the skin graft means you'll not be able to take anything but clear liquids by mouth for a while." He pauses. Dr. Jones knows the question that's coming.

"How long?" I scrawl across my tablet.

"Probably about four weeks, Marcus. I'm sorry, but for this procedure to have the best chance of success, we're going to need to rely only on your feeding tube for at least a month."

I am too stunned to speak. *A month?* It was just last week that I'd begun to eat milkshakes and creamy soup. Both have to be injected into my mouth with a syringe. Eating isn't high on my priority list, but a little flavor helps the hours pass. Now? That would all be taken away.

"Since you have a J tube, we'll keep pumping the Ensure and Magna-Cal into your intestine, but this means your stomach is going to be empty for a month. You'll get all your nutrition, but you're going to feel hunger pangs."

Still I sit, too shell-shocked to answer.

"We'll do the procedure tomorrow, Engels, and I'll be out to see you when Marcus goes to the recovery room," Dr. Jones says to my parents. He closes his chart and turns to me. "Any questions, Marcus?"

I shake my head. I cannot even summon the strength to write.

"How about you all, any questions?" he says to my parents.

"Yeah," my dad says. "The nurses are swabbing Marc's mouth with antiseptic mouthwash a couple times per day. Will that hurt the skin graft?"

"Not at all. In fact, I'll prescribe the same thing to help the surgical area heal. Just remind the nurse doing the cleaning to be extra careful around the grafted area. Any other questions?"

"You said only clear liquids by mouth. So, the milk-shakes and eggnog and soup are out of the question?" my mom asks, knowing this is going to be tough on me, physically AND emotionally.

"Unfortunately, yes. Clear liquids don't tend to stick to areas, but dairy based drinks do. If the food or drink sticks to the surgical area, it runs a higher chance of infection. As sensitive as this area is, any infection whatsoever could render the entire procedure a failure. I'm sorry, but this is just too important to Marcus' future oral health to allow anything beside clear liquids. Any other questions?"

"Just one," Dad says. "Once the four weeks are up, he can start to have only the milk based liquids again?"

"Oh, no!" Dr. Jones says, a bit of excitement in his voice. "After four weeks, he can have anything he can tolerate. Mashed potatos, yogurt, pudding – it doesn't just have to be liquids."

Well, a tiny glimmer of hope, but it'll take a month until we get to that point. Well, I went nearly a month without eating anything at all, so I can do it again. Thing is, that month of not eating was spent in a haze of pain killers. Now? I'm a lot more conscious… and sober. This will, without a doubt, be one hell of a month.

"If that's all the questions, I'll bid you good night. See you in pre-op tomorrow morning, Marcus," Dr. Jones says. He shakes my hand, then the hands of my parents. Then, he's gone.

If the patient has no medical background, explanations, even when thorough, may feel like drinking from a fire hose. There is so, SO much information coming at a patient; doctor's orders, nurses' reports, vital signs, medications… all this while the patient is most likely uncomfortable and on pain killers. It's a lot to sort out.

Stopping every so often to ask, "Do you have any questions so far?" gives the patient an opportunity to absorb info at their pace. You can give the most detailed, thorough explanations on earth with diagrams and arrows on color glossy photographs, but if the patient isn't with you, all that explanation goes to waste.

Remember, the hospital, the doctor's office, the nursing home, the rehab center – all these are YOUR place of employment. The information there is YOUR field of expertise. Your patient, on the other hand, comes into many medical situations ignorant of their own care. The more information they can understand, the more empowered the patient will feel and the faster their recovery.

CHAPTER 14

Pharmacological Confusion

The scrape of the metal hooks overhead tells me someone has just entered my makeshift cell.

Here we go again, I think. It's surgery day… again. Feels like the last one was just yesterday. Now, I'm back in pre-op. The temperature is cool, the room busy and hurried and I am nervous. When the metal hooks scrape their hello, I cross my fingers. I hope it's Dr. Jones. I'm wrong.

"Hi there," says a male voice. He gives a cursory nod to my parents, then comes to my bed. "I'm Dr. Franklin and I'll be your anesthesiologist today." He shakes my hand. "I'm just going to start with a little Vercet and Lovenox." He reaches above my head and a few IV tubes dangle at my shoulder. A slight beeping begins overhead. A motor begins to turn. Something electrical starts up.

"I'll be back in a few minutes and we'll take you down to the operating room."

The metal hooks scrape open, then closed. My body begins to feel heavy. I relax into the feeling… but, *Wait! What AM I feeling? Is this the drugs he just gave? Is this supposed to be happening?* Fear grips me. Uncertainty and nerves rear their ugly heads. *What if this isn't right? What if I'm dying? What if I'm having a heart attack? What if he gave me the wrong medication?* The questions pepper my brain. The heavy, warm feeling moves through me, my muscles feel weak and tired. I wish I could slip further into the feeling, but I don't know if I should... *what am I supposed to do?*

Here are three words you may not know: Charlais. Baldassarre. Palahniuk.

Would you like any of these injected into your body? Likely no... for a variety of reasons. The first of which is simply because they're unknown.

Here's the scoop: Charlais is a breed of cattle that my grandfather raised. Baldassarre is the first name of a 15th century evil governor of Bologna, Italy. Palahniuk is the last name of one of my favorite authors, Chuck Palahniuk.

Now that you have perspective and definitions, you can safely answer that no, if you have an IV, you do NOT want any of these injected into your body, right?

Medications often have difficult names. Many patients know the basics of pharmacy drugs: antibiotics, narcotics, anti-inflammatory. But it's simply wrong to assume the patient knows what you're talking about when listing off medications.

Lovenox and Vercet? Those words are probably as foreign to the patient as Baldassarre is to you. Comfort your patient by explaining what each medication is used for. Even though I'd been given Vercet, a drug intended to help me relax, I couldn't actually relax because I didn't know what to expect. Instead of simply naming the medication, take an extra couple seconds to explain what that drug is going to do.

CHAPTER 15

Your Connection Is Not Your Patient's Biggest Concern

"My uncle went blind from diabetes, Marcus," says my nurse on duty. I nod. That's about all I can muster. It's about all I care to muster, too.

"Yeah, he'd been diabetic since childhood, but when he was in his 40's, he started losing his sight. For a long time, he would just cope with what he had. He didn't drive at night any more, but he still did during the day. Maybe he shouldn't have, but he did. Then, when he was around 50, it really started to go."

I need morphine. And some ice chips. And I'd like to have some time with my Mom and Dad.

"When he finally went totally blind, he got trained as a piano tuner. He used to get his books on tape and had all kinds of little devices to help him out. I remember he had this thing we called the Rattlesnake. It was a buzzer with two long prongs that he'd hang over a coffee cup. It looked like a rattlesnake's head and fangs when the venom was being drained out. Anyway, that thing would buzz to let him know the coffee cup was full."

I still need morphine. I still want ice chips. I still want my parents nearby.

"Oh, and the other thing he had was this special radio. It ran on different frequencies or something, I'm not sure. But it was really big and it broadcasted stuff for blind people. I think it was housed in a regular radio station, but ran on different radio waves. Anyway, they'd always read the paper from beginning to end, the grocery store advertisements and everything. I hope you can get one of those, Marcus!"

I hope I can get some morphine. And ice chips. And my parents...

Please, PLEASE don't get me wrong. I'm a huge advocate of finding commonalities between patient and caregiver. However, those commonalities should be used to make your patient more comfortable and connected with his/her care. This nurse had her heart in the right place. Heck, she even had good information for me, but at that point, I wasn't asking for her to pontificate on everything she knew about blindness. We had bigger fish to fry. Yet, she was still serving me sardines about a long dead uncle who happened to share the same disability.

Finding commonalities with patients IS important, but it's not more important than their comfort. Unless it deals directly with their care, it doesn't help a patient to know how much you know. Until the relationship is established, keep the common life experiences to a couple of sentences. If the patient further engages you, go for it! But keep the connections to compliments and cursory comments. Remember, your patient's biggest concern is his/her well being, not your connection.

CHAPTER 16

"Screw Your Policy"

"Marcus, you have some visitors," says my nurse on duty. I give her the thumbs up, just coming out of a deep sleep. I make a writing motion with my hand. She places my tablet across my lap and I fumble for the pen.

"*What time is it?*" I write out.

"Ten 'til nine," she says, sounding a little miffed. "Visiting hours end in 10 minutes, Marcus."

I shrug, a motion that says I don't care about what posted visiting hours are, I want to see my friends. Everyone knows that. Everyone knows that if I'm asleep, awake, hurting, doing physical therapy, eating, drinking, thinking, sitting – whatever I'm doing, it will stop when I have visitors. I feed off information from the outside world. People, objects, stories – anything outside this hospital helps me think that maybe, someday, I'll be back in the world.

"*Who is it?*" I write again, paying no mind to her report that visiting hours are almost over.

"I think one said he was your roommate," she says. "There are three guys, at least."

I give another thumbs up.

"Okay, I'll get them, but keep it short, okay, Marcus?" I give her a dismissive wave.

They are, in fact, my roommates. Two of them, at least, with another guy who lived across the hall. Three and a half hours by car. Nearly 200 miles. Visitors, friends, guys who were cutting their teeth on college at the same time as me. They'll continue to – I won't. At least, not for a while.

They gather around my bed, shake my hand, tell me they miss me at school. I communicate as best I can, scrawling everything out on paper. It's a slow, cumbersome way to talk. After half an hour, the nurse re-appears.

"Hey guys, she says. "Visiting hours were supposed to be over at 9 p.m." She isn't angry, isn't forceful, just stating the rules.

The guys all prepare to leave, not wanting to infringe on hospital policy. I motion for the nurse to come near the bed.

"Why do they have to leave?" I scrawl.

"It's hospital policy that visiting hours end at 9 p.m., Marcus," she says. Again, not angry, just stating the rules.

"Screw that policy," I scrawl. *"We're not disturbing anyone, are we?"*

"No, you're being quiet, I'm just telling you the policy." She states.

"These guys came a long way to see me. I'm not kicking them out now."

The nurse pauses, contemplating. My roommates shuffle nervously. They've spent all evening driving, only to arrive at some pre-determined hour that doesn't really fit a college guy's schedule. That long of a drive for a 30 minute chit chat session seems wasteful... and disrespectful.

"Okay, you're right, Marcus," she says, resigning that there's no hope to get them to leave. "I'll close the door to the hallway so you guys won't have to whisper. If you need anything, just hit the nurse call light, okay?" I give a thumbs up.

⟨⟩

Unfortunately, when people hear the words, "Our policy," they may perceive it as a challenge. They're likely to see that statement as the point from which the other party will not budge. When that line is drawn in the sand, tempers can flare. Patients may want something, but they're told "the policy" won't allow their request to be filled.

If a patient's request is dangerous or harmful, that's a golden opportunity to explain, not only the policy, but why it is in place.

Here's an example: Let's say a patient wants a family member to bring them a six pack of beer. Rather than simply stating the hospital's policy about alcohol on the premises, explain how mixing alcohol with the patient's current medications can cause respiratory arrest, seizures, whatever the real danger is. By educating the patient, you offer them an opportunity to return home with knowledge that might save their life.

Visiting hours can be sticky. If a long-term patient needs visitors (like I so desperately needed friends around), there can be confusion over how to handle the situation. On one hand, the health care pro knows the patient thrives off visits. On the other, these visits come outside of visiting hours. What to do?

Your author has never (and will never) tell you it is okay to go against hospital policy. I will, however, express how much I appreciated my nurses making individualized decisions based on my situation. When there was no harm to myself nor the other patients on the floor, it gave me so much comfort and help when the visiting hours were extended a little bit. But again, each case, each individual patient, each scenario needs to be evaluated on its own merit.

CHAPTER 17

"You Can't Expect Miracles The First Day"

"Hey, Marcus! What's going on, dude?" A voice booms from overhead. I've been asleep, but this thundering male voice has pulled me from slumberland back into here and now land. Even though sleep is precious, I'm intrigued. Not only is this guy booming, but he's also smiling.

I reach for my tablet and pencil, but before I can find them, a massive paw of a hand grabs mine. The hand pumps mine in a shake. The grip is so powerful that it hurts my bruised arm, but I smile on the inside. Whoever this guy is, he's not going to baby me.

"I'm Dennis Fuller," he says, dropping my hand and shoving my tablet onto my lap. "I'm a speech pathologist, dude. I'm going to try to get you talking again, okay?" I nod.

Talking? Really? For weeks, the trach has kept me silent. Worse than that is the possibility that something in my vocal mechanism might be injured... permanently. I've mentally explored the idea of living as a blind mute. These possibilities aren't pretty.

"How?" I scrawl out.

"How? How, you ask, dude?" Dennis booms out, totally excited to be in this moment. I nod feebly.

"Well, this isn't rocket science, so I'll tell ya! I have here in my hand a small plastic tube. Here, check it out!" He shoves a small, circular tube attached to a string into my palm. I roll it around a few times between my fingers. It's unimpressive, just a plastic cylinder. Nothing special.

"You have this trach in your throat. It helps you breathe, but it lets your voice take a vacation. This talking trach will force your body to do its natural job. That is, it'll push your voice through your vocal mechanism and that'll create audible sound, just like your voice worked before. Ready to try it?"

I nod, but quickly grab at my tablet. *"Will it hurt?"* I write.

"Nah, not a bit! I promise ya, dude!"

With that, I feel a few fingers at my throat. A tiny, almost inaudible click sounds.

"There! Done!" Dennis says, stepping back to admire his handiwork.

"Okay, dude," he booms. "Let's take it for a test drive! Wanna do some counting? Repeat after me: One, two, three, four."

I do as he says, but as soon as "One" comes out, I stop. I sound like the speech impaired ghost of a drunken sailor. Just horrible. "One" comes out as "hun." A bewildered and horrified look crosses my face.

"Don't sweat it, man, okay?" Dennis says, seeing my concern. "Look, your voice has been chilling at Club Med for like three weeks. It's time for it to get back to work.

But to do that, it's gotta get back in shape with practice, okay?" I nod.

"Cool. Wanna try counting again?" I do. It's only slightly better; like, maybe the ghost had an hour to sober up. As soon as I finish, Dennis says, "Awesome! Do it again!" His enthusiasm is like a little kid watching a circus performer do some unthinkable task. Contagious enthusiasm, I think, as I begin again.

"Hun,who, heree, hore."

"Excellent!" Dennis says excitedly.

"Is Aw-hul," I slur. Dennis understands perfectly. Even through the slurring, the weak vocal inflection, the swollen and paralyzed lips, he still hears the complaint: "It's awful."

"No, no it's not, dude! This is exactly what we expect after a couple weeks of no talking. It'll get better, I promise! You'll just have to practice. Just wait – you'll see!"

"Hrully?" I gasp.

"Yes, really. I mean, it's going to take a little time. You can't expect miracles the first day, but with a little practice, you'll be like... wait, who's your favorite singer?"

"Honnie Ash," I blurt.

"Yeah, dude, you're not going to sound like Johnny Cash today. Actually, you're probably never going to sound like the man in black, but that's just because he's cooler than we normal guys, right?" I give a little huff of a chuckle.

"Just keep practicing. No miracles the first day, but you'll be talking great soon, okay, dude?"

Realistic expectations were key. Had Dr. Fuller told me I'd be a Harry Connick Jr. crooner overnight, it would have been a lie. What he promised me was, if I followed the process of practice, I had some level of control over how my voice would heal.

Many patients will grab onto what they want to believe, not what the health care pro actually says. Dennis made it clear that this might be a long haul, not an instantaneous change. He was right… after three weeks of not using any part of the body, to think it'd snap back into perfection immediately would be foolish. To give me the realistic facts not only gave me the truth of the situation, but it gave me a plan for how to improve.

CHAPTER 18

"Come Undone?"

There are three long slabs of tape above my wrist. An inch apart, these three sections secure the tube that attaches to the IV in the back of my right hand. Saline and morphine and heavy narcotics and heavier antibiotics are shot into this mess, only to be delivered to my system.

Right now, more than anything, *I want it out*. The tape itches something fierce. At the back of my hand where the IV connects with my skin, at the three sites where the tape holds down the tube, and the tube itself, sticky rubber yanks at the hair on my arm. When the follicles are pulled, it's like nails on a chalkboard. Worse than nails. Nails and glass and copper pipes and teeth, all scraping into a Satanic symphony. The tape burns, itches, teases my skin. *I want it gone – now.*

With my left hand, I slowly, purposefully begin to dismantle this torture device. The highest site, the tape across my forearm, is the first to go. With an intentional pull, I brace for the hair to be yanked out at the root. A sharp intake of breath accompanies the action. Next section of tape, same process. Third verse, same as the first.

The IV tube dangles from my wrist like a dead snake. I begin to pull at the tape around the IV. This is harder – a lot harder. Instead of single slabs of tape, this is a pile. Layers upon layers. The going is slower, more deliberate. After the first layer, I'm beginning to get a rhythm. A few more minutes and this wretched stuff will be off. My skin can breathe again. Then, a soft knock at the door.

"Hey kiddo," Barb says, striding in. "How ya doing?"

She reaches my bed. I pause. I know she doesn't approve. She spent nearly 20 minutes getting the IV arranged and secured when she first started her shift. Now? Her patient has destroyed her handiwork.

"Oh no," Barb says, but there's no emergency, no condemnation.

"This came undone. Sorry about that, Marcus... I'll fix it so this won't happen again." I nod, claiming no responsibility. Barb also places none on me.

She steps across the room, grabs a roll of tape from her supplies and returns.

"Your skin seems aggravated around where the tape was. I'll clean that off so it's more comfortable, okay, Marcus?" I nod again, still not speaking.

I know I've done something that wasn't in the plan. I know I've caused more work for Barb. I know the IV is important to be kept in place... and I haven't cared. I've just been so, so focused on the irritation that all I've wanted is to get it off my skin – now!

Barb uses an alcohol swab to remove the sticky residue from the tape site. The alcohol feels cool and clean. "Let's give this a few minutes to dry and give your skin some recovery time, okay?" Again, I nod.

Barb hangs around, not checking vitals, not cleaning me, not doing anything but hanging out with her patient. Our conversation is sparse – I'm still aggravated at my discomfort. Barb seems to sense this and gives me an extra long reprieve before ripping another section of tape from the roll.

"I'll cut these pieces of tape in half," she says, pressing the first reinforcement across the IV tube. "It'll still be as secure as earlier, but there won't be as much tape so it won't hurt your skin. That sound okay?"

Again, I nod, still not speaking. We have this mutual understanding; whatever has happened, it's in the past. From now on, I'll be taken care of even better.

⌒

Notice Barb's words: "This came undone." Who is to blame? Not her patient – THAT is key. Even though it was me who consciously tried to remove the aggravation, Barb isn't worried about the wrong I did. She's also not worried about assigning blame. She objectifies the negative, making it sound as though tape, tubes and dressing spontaneously remove themselves.

Do they? Not in this case: the direct goal was to keep it secure. I undermined that effort and nearly caused the destruction of the plan. Yet, did Barb see the damage and ask, "What'd you do this for?" Not even close. She knew that sort of accusation and observation would put me on the defensive. The goal again? Keep the area safe and secure. The secondary goal? Keep the patient comfortable while goal #1 is going on.

Does assigning blame help in any way? Does lecturing a heavily medicated patient about their bad behavior make them want to act better? Patients are in such a vulnerable state that addition of guilt and wrongdoing is less than helpful – it's just plain hurtful.

CHAPTER 19

Help Patients Retain Modesty

Eight of my buddies gather around my bed. Just three days ago, I regained the ability to speak, thanks to a talking trach installed by my speech pathologist. My voice is still shaky and slurred, but at least I can communicate again verbally... sorta.

"Dude, Engel," one friend says, "We were coming in through the lobby and there were just tons of hot nurses around! I mean tons, dude! I'll move in and be your roommate and I'll get some of them to give us sponge baths!"

We all laugh at this. It's just me and the guys, same as always. Well, almost.

There's a knock at the door. As Barb enters the room, the laughter dies down. It's almost like we got caught laughing in class – only Barb isn't like a teacher giving out reprimands. In fact, she loves to see her favorite patient laughing it up with the boys.

Hey guys!" Barb exclaims as she walks up to my bed. "Geez, it's like a locker room in here! Marcus, I'm going to have to be sure you don't overdose on testosterone!"

"No need to worry about that with Engel," one of the guys says. "He's so full of estrogen he'll probably start his period any minute now!" Everyone laughs, me included, but I can't let a good-natured teasing go unpunished. I point in the direction where the voice just came, then flip him the bird.

This is the kind of male bonding and teasing torture that typically goes on with teenage guys. The uninitiated would think this mean-spirited – not Barb! She has two teenage boys of her own. She's probably heard this kind of stuff around her house, too.

"All right, gentlemen," Barb says. "I need you all to step over here by the window so I can do some treatments for Marc." The guys, all eight of them, obey and move toward the south window. Barb swings my TV around to face the guys. "You guys wanna watch ESPN while I do some wound treatment for Marc?" she asks. "Hell, yeah!" comes back their response, almost in a profane unison. Barb hits the buttons and the sound of the highlight film fills the air.

"Also, if you look out the far left side of the window, you can see Busch Stadium and the Arch," She says, turning her attention back to her patient.

Barb grabs three pillows and stands them against the bed rail on my left. Then, she positions herself near my left hip.

"I've gotta change the dressing at your abdominal wound, then flush out your J tube," Barb says in a low breath.

My abdominal incision is above my navel, but the other incisions are in the crease of my leg and crotch. Normally, Barb would simply draw the curtain so no one from the hallway could see in, then lift my sheets and robe. Now, with my buds here, she piles first the blanket, then the sheet, in tall mountains of fabric. One is mounded up on my belly and chest, the other just south of my crotch. No one to the right of my bed, and Barb is blocking everyone's view to the left.

She quickly flushes my J tube, then changes the dressing over my abdominal scar. The procedures take no more than five minutes. All the while, Barb only speaks to me. She quickly tucks my robe back into place. When I'm covered again, she lays the blanket flat across my mid-section. Pillows are replaced under each arm, the sheets are folded and slid back onto another holder. When she's finished, Barb moves to the right side of my bed. She speaks to the guys again, telling them thanks for coming to visit me. "And keep it down, okay? I don't want any of the other patients calling security to break up any parties, guys!" Everyone laughs – including Barb and me.

$$\smile\!\!\!\!\!\supset$$

Even though these guys and I had played football together for the past four years, and even though we'd all probably been in the locker room showers at the same time, and even though we'd probably all jumped out of a pickup together to take a piss along some dirt road, Barb instinctively knew I wouldn't want to be exposed. There, in front of my friends. Like this.

She used everything in her power to help my friends get their focus on something else (the view out the window and the television.) Next, she blocked their view with pillows, sheets, blankets and her own body. Positioning herself between the guys and me, her body was the natural barrier to hide my nudity.

Third, once she began performing her tasks, she spoke only to me. This helped create the dynamic that this was "Barb and Marcus" time and that others needed to respect our privacy. Plus, before she ever started to do my dressings, she had all her bandages, gauze and ointment there, ready and laid out. Her procedures were able to be accomplished in mere minutes due to pre-planning.

Patients in the hospital give up so, SO much modesty. They get used to having their naked body exposed to the rest of their caregivers. They become all too accustomed to having a nurse or tech wipe their butt, check their foley, open their shirt to reveal a breast while listening to their heart with a stethoscope. For me, Barb gave me the ability to keep some degree of privacy, while not forcing my friends out into the waiting room.

What can you do to help your patient retain their modesty? Sheets, pillows, distractions – anything you can do to keep your patient's private parts from being exposed to the world will help them feel more like they are in control of their own body.

CHAPTER 20

Creating Confidence And Trust With The Patient's Family

I am fucking sick to death of everything. The pain, the doctors, the constant interruptions, the inability to eat, the never-ending beeps of my monitors, the volume of passers-by in the hallways, the dull roar of the TV across the hall, the quiet tone of the nurse call light flashing on above other doors. I am angry, I'm powerless and I'm full of hate. Anyone within reach of my bed is going to get an earful of profanity and anger.

"Do you want some water?" Mom asks tentatively.

I exhale in frustration. "No, I don't want any damned water!" I slur in a yell.

"Is there anything I can do to help?" she asks, tears welling up in her eyes. Her tears only add fuel to the fire. I'm tired of people feeling sorry for me. I'm tired of being poked and prodded. I'm tired of being in this room. I just want to be left alone – for a long, long time.

"Yes, you can leave me be and get out of here!" I'm so hurt and I just want to hurt everyone around me. Violence, insults, curses – I don't care. I just want to lash out.

There's a soft knock at the door. "Can I come in?" Barb asks. Even Barb is subject to my foul mood. I give a frustrated sigh and wave my hand in a "What choice do I have?" motion.

"Rough day, buddy?" Barb asks, coming up to the edge of my bed.

"It wouldn't be if people would just leave me the hell alone!" I spit out.

"I'm sorry, Marc," Barb says, truly sympathetic. I can almost hear the compassionate glance she gives my parents. "You've been doing so good for so long, Marc, you were about due for a bad day."

I scowl, the right side of my face pinches. The left stays unmoving. This pisses me off, all over again. Barb gives my hand a sympathetic squeeze.

"Mom and Dad," she says, turning to them, but still holding my hand, "Why don't you guys take a little break? I think Marc could use a little time on his own. I'll be right here if he needs anything, but for now, why don't you guys go get a cup of coffee?"

The uninitiated may see this as Barb shooing off my parents with a polite dismissal. Negative. Barb had already established the relationship with me and, thereby, with my parents. She worked to fulfill the patient's request, but comforted my parents by reassuring them that she's still here, that their son was safe and would be taken care of.

Furthermore, she showed that this kind of emotion is normal and expected. When the patient's family trusts in the caregiver, the patient will, too.

CHAPTER 21

"This Won't Hurt A Bit"

Today has been a bad day. That's putting it mildly. Picture a loan shark with two huge goons. One goon grabs me and holds my arms. The other, on the shark's command, punches me in the stomach. Every time a right lands in my belly, I let out a "Ooof!" as the air expels from my lungs. Then, as soon as I begin to breathe again, a left hand clocks me across my jaw. Right, belly, left, face. Right, left, belly, face. Over and over and over again.

There are no goons. There is no loan shark. There is no one holding my hands behind my back. There is just routine. No one purposefully tries to hurt me, but there are things that need to be done.

I only slept a few minutes last night. Hallucinations popped into my brain every time I'd drift off. I'd wake with a start, the sudden movement tearing at the empty places in my chest where ribs used to be. At dawn, I drift off into a restless sleep. Thirty minutes later, there's a quiet knock at the door. The breakfast cart. The person from dietary moves some things on my table, then places the tray down next to my stereo. I imagine I can smell the food. Eggs, bacon, oatmeal, pancakes. In reality, only the strongest scents are noticed by my olfactory system. Air freshener, the smell of my own waste as I sit on a commode, the stench of cigarette smoke on a caregiver. This breakfast doesn't truly have smell that I can detect – it's only wishful thinking. I don't want the food, I just want to sleep. And I cannot. The person from dietary exits the room. I take deep breaths, trying to relax back into unconsciousness.

Just as I begin to drift off, there's a knock at the door.

"Hey buddy, it's Barb," says a chipper voice. I don't feel chipper. I just want to rest.

"Hey," I say, sounding slurred and sleepy, even to my own ear.

"You sleepy?" Barb asks.

"Yeah," I say.

"I'm sorry, buddy," Barb says, genuinely feeling sympathy for my discomfort. I nod.

"My shift ends in an hour. I was wondering if you want to try to use the commode before I take off?"

I nod. I don't really want to, but I'd rather get this task out of the way. And God knows who'll be my nurse when Barb's shift ends. Whoever it is, they won't be as good, as gentle, as friendly, as sympathetic as Barb.

We begin the arduous process of getting me out of bed. Turn on my side, scoot to the edge of the bed, rest, legs off the bed. Holding my arms out while Barb helps pull me into a sitting position. Rest. Deep breaths. Gather strength. She places a walker in front of me. My "good" leg touches the floor. Hands on the grips of the walker. Steady, steady. Barb faces me and grabs under my armpits. Slowly, carefully, I stand. Stop, breathe, re-group. We turn to the left, Barb places the commode behind me. We ease my naked rear onto this adult potty chair. By the time I'm seated and solid, there's sweat on my forehead.

"I'm going to give you some privacy for a few minutes, okay, Marcus?" I nod. I do my business. I try to wipe as best I can. I fail. I am so hurt, so unsteady, so helpless that I cannot even wipe my own ass. My face scrunches in anguish. I cannot cry – crying will just hurt even more. *Breathe, Engel, breathe.*

Barb returns, helps me get clean, changes the bed sheets and we reverse the process. The entire session takes nearly 40 minutes.

Back in bed, I'm ready to sleep. Barb bids me good-bye and says she'll see me tonight. I give a little wave. I sleep.

Another knock at the door. A new nurse. I've been asleep maybe five minutes, maybe ten. Either way, not enough.

"I'm Cheryl, Marcus. I'll be your nurse on duty today." I nod, just wanting her to leave so I can sleep.

"I need to change the dressing on your road rash," she says. I don't want this, I don't want to move, I don't want the pain of ripping off bandages, yanking hair, having to roll to my side. I don't want any of it. Still, I comply.

Roll, disrobe, expose my thighs, my butt, my back. The ripping of tape, the pain of hair being pulled out by its roots. Alcohol across large sections of my ass and back. Time to let it dry. Polysporin across the wounds. Gauze and tape and bandages to cover them again. Robe back in place. Slowly roll back onto my back. Cheryl leaves. I want to sleep – need to sleep.

Back into unconsciousness again. Again, a knock at the door. *Are you freaking kidding?* I think.

"Mr. Engel? I'm Dan, one of your friendly neighborhood vampires. Dr. Jones has ordered some blood drawn."

I nod, frustrated as all hell. I just want to sleep, for God's sake!

"Do you have an arm you'd prefer me to draw from?" he asks.

"Yeah, yours!" I blurt out. He's taken aback. He says nothing. I point at my right arm and place a finger at the crook of my elbow.

His demeanor is now subdued. "I need to take four vials," he says, wiping an alcohol swab across my arm. I nod again.

"Just get it over with," I mumble.

The needle hits my vein. I feel the cold metal puncture my skin. The pain is enormous. *Why does it hurt so much?* I have blood drawn almost every day – why does this one hurt so much more? I gasp in a huge breath of air and face my head to the sky.

"One down, three to go," he says, and I hear something plastic click.

My gut clenches with the pain, my nerves scream for release. I notice I'm holding my breath and I begin to exhale. *In, out, in, out.*

"Almost done, this is the last one," Dan says, working as fast as he can. My head and neck begin to shiver with exertion. *Why does this freaking hurt so much? It's just blood being drawn... why does it feel like he's chopping off my arm?*

Finally, Dan says, "There, done." My body relaxes into a heap. I am too drained to speak. I don't even acknowledge him when he says, "Thanks, Marcus. Have a good day." I take one breath. Then two. Then three. I'm so exhausted I can't sleep. But, I try to relax. Breathe, count sheep, count backwards, relaxation exercises, visualization. Peaceful thoughts. Finally, I begin to feel my body unwind.

Like a police interrogation, another knock comes at the door.

"You sleepin', Brother?" says the familiar voice of my Dad.

"I'm trying to," I angrily blurt out. I don't want to get upset, I don't want to hurt any more, I don't want to do anything but sleep.

"Okay, we'll be quiet," My mom says. And they will. They love me, they don't want me to hurt.

I drift back into unconsciousness. This time, though, there are no interruptions. My parents run interference for me. Housekeepers come to the door. "Later," my mom whispers and shakes her head, waving them off. Dietary comes with the lunch tray. Mom points to an open chair where they can leave the tray. Her whispers tell the delivery person to keep it down. Nurses arrive, again and again and again. While they have tasks to complete, my need for sleep is overwhelming. Maternal instinct tells my mother this, too.

Finally, there is a knock at the door that can't be ignored. I hear the clatter of a cart being wheeled in.

"Marcus? I'm Darren and I'm going to do an EKG on you, okay?" I shake my head furiously, not wanting to deal with any more hurt today.

"No?" Darren asks, curious. He pauses.

"I don't want it to hurt!" I blurt out, not caring at this point if I'm rude or not.

"Oh, Marcus, this won't hurt a bit! All I do is attach a couple of pads to your chest. The test only takes a couple minutes and you won't feel a thing – I promise you, this won't hurt a bit!"

After such a horrible day of interruptions, painful procedures and no sleep, the last thing I wanted was to hurt more. The assurance of "This won't hurt a bit!" was so genuine that I became at ease. While I didn't know what an EKG was, what I wanted most was to rest without additional pain.

As always, procedures in the hospital are commonplace to you, the health care professional. But patients often don't know an EKG from a CBC, an ultrasound from an injection. And really, many times patients won't care. Their biggest concern is: Will this hurt?

After being hospitalized and undergoing so, so many procedures, I became punch drunk with how many "things" needed to be done to me. I ultimately stopped resisting all things, just giving up fighting. Every time there was something new that needed to be injected, extracted, removed, added, etc. to my body, I had just one question: Will this hurt?

Patients may or may not care what procedure you have to do. Even if you explain what an EKG or a CBC is, they may still be confused. But everyone, EVERYONE cares if the procedure will hurt. The more you can prepare your patient for what to expect in the procedure, the better care you are providing.

Chapter 22

Behold, I Stand At The Door And Knock

I am feeling very, very poor. Not sickly, but impoverished. And very out of control. My life has been reduced to this room, this bed, this pillow and a few items on my bedside table. A small stereo, a couple CDs and a stuffed animal. This robe? Not mine. These tubes in my arms? Not mine. These stockings on my legs, this pillow and case, this bed, these sheets, this TV, this room – none of it is mine.

And my body? Also not mine. There are needles, tubes, metal implants and incisions in my body. Not mine. I don't want them, but they've invaded my body. I no longer own the body into which I was born. The senses I was born with? Gone... or, at least, partially gone. Sight? Not any more. Hearing? Maybe half of what it should be. Smell, taste, touch? All diminished in some form or another. Nothing is mine – not even me.

In the midst of my self loathing, there comes a knock at the door. Then another. Then another. *Knock, knock, knock.*

I take a deep breath. I don't want to have visitors. I'm in the midst of a pity party and I'm the honored guest. The knocks come again. Slowly, I turn my head and look to the door.

"Yeah?" I say to the person in the hallway.

"It's Barb, Marc. Can I come in?"

⟲⟶

Yours truly received a minor in criminal justice studies from Missouri State University. God knows what I was thinking to get my degree in CJS, but hey, here we are. Anyway, one thing from my classes translates well to patient care.

During one of my semesters, there was a national news story about a prisoner being beaten to death in prison. The news pointed out (almost gleefully, I might add) that the prisoner who'd done the beating did so because the deceased sat on his bed. Beaten to death… for copping a squat on a bed that didn't belong to him.

One of my professors shared this story with us and explained some things about prison culture. To understand the value of one's bed, you've got to take a step inside the cell and the skin of a prisoner. Every earthly possession they own is taken away when they're incarcerated. Personal items – gone. Then, they're assigned to a cell. Apartment, house, trailer, whatever they used to live in – gone. Replaced by a room the size of a walk in closet. A toilet in the room with no bathroom doors, walls, or windows. Personal space? Gone. This tiny cell houses not one, but two inmates. Sometimes three. Each prisoner gets a bed or a cot. It's theirs. No one else's. With everything else stripped away, that bed is their only possession. And many prisoners will protect their bed with the ferocity of a mother bear keeping her newborn cubs safe.

Now, replace "prisoner" with "patient." Identical situations? Not exactly, but there are similarities. The patient isn't in their own abode; they're likely sharing a room with another patient. Many people have never slept in the same room as another adult once they left home. Or, if they did, it may have been with a spouse. Patients are completely out of their element, at best. At worst, they may even feel trapped.

Barb seemed to sense this. She wanted to respect my space. She seemed to know that my body no longer truly belonged to me. Nor did my bed, my room, nothing. And her solution was to give me the control over who entered. Would I ever tell Barb she couldn't come in? Never! But just having that power back gave me some sense of control.

Consider giving three knocks before walking in on a patient. Your patients probably already feel out of control, and you have a golden opportunity to empower them in their own environment.

CHAPTER 23

Personalize
Positive Progress

"Can I get a look at this leg?" Barb asks, tapping the toes of my left foot.

"Sure thing," I say, flipping off the sheets and blankets onto my other leg. This process used to be a lot more painful. At first, my leg was just scraped and bloody and bruised. Then, both legs went into traction, hanging above my bed like the legs of some untalented skier. After the traction, my right leg was fine, but the left still needed some work – a lot of work. Next procedure attached an external fixator to the left leg. Pins still protruded from three, four, five points between the knee and the ankle.

On the inside of my left leg, a thick metal bar was attached to the head of each pin that stuck out from the skin. Picture the rude hardware of a crowbar attached to some ultra sensitive looking medical implants; like a farmer plowing a field in a tuxedo. They just didn't look right together. Then, off with the external fixator and a single 20 inch rod called an IM nail was inserted into my kneecap and pounded down the bone all the way to the ankle. The left leg was then encased in a plaster cast.

Strange, prior to the crash, I'd never broken a single bone. And with all the other damage done to my body, this was the first time I'd ever had a cast. Now, the cast, too, was gone and my leg lay naked and shriveled. My muscles had such severe atrophy that they looked like they belonged to a 10 year old girl... a tall, hairy 10 year old girl.

Barb has been with me throughout the healing process on the leg. While this is the plastic surgery floor and orthopedics aren't usually what she treats, Barb had faithfully done wound care over my knee and at the pin sites for weeks now. And finally, FINALLY, the biggest wound of all, the giant strawberry covering my patella, was starting to heal.

Barb tucks the sheet around my leg. I feel cool air below the waist for the first time in several hours.

"Hey! You can't imagine how good you've got this looking, Marcus!"Barb exclaims. "Really?" I ask, intrigued.

"Totally! It's even shrunk in size since yesterday! You're doing a really great job getting this healed up!" She gathers the alcohol and Polysporin for this session of wound care.

"Um, you know I really haven't done anything to make this heal better, right?" I ask, not wanting to take credit where credit isn't due.

"Not true, buddy, not true! Sure, you heal fast naturally, but you've certainly played a role here. So many times, I'll get patients who will keep picking at their wounds – you haven't done that. And you always let me treat it with alcohol. I know that hurts, but you ignore the hurt and allow it to be cleaned."

I shrug.

"And ya know what else, Marcus? It's real tough to heal wounds on the knee. That area bends and re-opens the wound every time you move your leg. You've done a great job at keeping your leg still, buddy."

"But I can't really even move my leg – it hurts too much to bend it."

"Well, however you've done it, you've got this wound almost healed completely!"

Always remember: patients are out of their element, potentially confused, drugged and may feel powerless. Barb's way of conversing made me feel as though several different positive things were going on: First, the wound is healing. Second, I was responsible for this healing. Third, no one BUT me could heal this area as well as I!

For any improvement, Barb gave me the accolades and credit. Did I really deserve that? Maybe, maybe not, but her way of talking to me made me feel like I was being proactive in my own care.

CHAPTER 24

Respect Your Patient's Time

Here we go again. Massive orderlies, the crack of my ribs as my sling bed is lifted skyward. The precarious rocking of the wheelchair as I'm lowered into it. The tucking of the sheets into the seat so they won't interfere with the wheels and gears. A nurse juggles tubes and oxygen tanks and IV poles onto my moving hospital room.

My shoulders are heavy. I slump forward. My abdominal muscles are just gone; gone with the rest of my muscles. I've dropped 50 pounds in a matter of weeks and my body looks like that of a prisoner in a concentration camp. I grab the arms of the wheel chair to steady my body as we move through the endless corridors of Barnes Hospital. Along the way, I take deep breaths and try, try to convince myself that this is a step forward. It's my first time out of my hospital room, other than being pushed in my bed. This wheelchair trip isn't fun – far from it. But it does make me feel like there's a forward motion to my life. Baby steps into something more normal; that is, if normalcy is ever even possible again.

We arrive at a new doctor's office. The secretary greets us and says, "The doctor will see you in just a few minutes."

This doctor apparently has patients who are more injured, more hurt, more precarious than I. I'm sarcastic and angry. I do not want to wait in the waiting room. This chair is uncomfortable; my heart beats loudly in my chest. We wait. And wait. And wait. My nurse gave a shot of morphine before we left. It's starting to wear off. I tense even more. And still, we wait. Names are called from the secretary's desk: MacIntyre, Gregory, Wells, Knight. More names are called. With each name, I grow a degree more angry. My ass screams in pain, the bedsores and road rash sting with a fiery ache. Still, we wait.

After what is nearly an hour, the secretary says, "Engel." I'm wheeled back into the exam room. Again, we wait. I am silent, too angry, too hurt, too frustrated to speak. The surgeon finally arrives. He seems hurried. He talks fast, he moves fast, he writes fast. He is unsafe. I need slow motions that will not jar my body. If he swings around on his stool, his knee will strike my leg and I will scream. I will scream to burst his eardrums. He has left me uncomfortable, worried and hurting. And now he is scaring me with these jackrabbit motions. He explains to my parents what he will do in the next surgery. He jots some notes and says he'll speak to my parents when I go to the recovery room. The doctor exits.

The orderly returns. The trip has been endless. Well over an hour, most of this time was spent sitting in the waiting room. Waiting. Waiting for a doctor to come in and look at me for three minutes. Time spent angry and frustrated I had to wait. Why couldn't he have come to my room? Why couldn't he have worked me in when I arrived? Why did I have to wait nearly an hour in the waiting room while not-so-injured patients went in before me? I'm so exhausted I want to cry. But I can't. Not yet. We still have to get me back into bed. Yet more pain and fear to an already endless day.

As a teenager, I used to get my hair cut about every three weeks. I'd swing into my stylist's chair, she'd give me a quick trim and I'd be on my merry way. She once explained how she estimates 30 minutes for every man's haircut, 45 for every woman's. Then, every several hours, the stylist would block off a 30 minute "cut" for no one. Just an empty buffer of time. Why?

Inevitably, one haircut would take longer than expected. When that would happen, it pushed all appointments back by half an hour. Or, maybe longer, depending on the cut. Instead of having her clients show up and wait for her to play catch up, she would budget in the time. All of this out of the simple respect for her client's time.

Picture this: What would happen if I'd arrived at the doctor's office and they were backed up... but, instead of leaving me sit in the waiting room, they'd apologized? "Marcus, I'm really sorry, but the doctor is running behind and it's going to be at least a half an hour." Would I have been aggravated? Sure, but at least I'd have known what I was getting into. And what if the office staff had the forethought to see this battered teenager in the waiting room and pulled some strings? What if they'd asked a patient before me (quietly), "The young man in the wheelchair is a patient here in the hospital and his appoint-

ment is after you. Would you mind switching appointment times with him? It shouldn't be more than 15 minutes?" Most any patient, seeing someone in such horrible shape, would happily switch places.

But, does this even need to be done? Why doesn't someone see a need, then do their best to fill it? Always communicate the situation to the patient. Then, work within your limitations to make it an easy transition for the patient.

Do what you can to respect your patient's time. Maybe even take a lesson from the sign posted on the secretary's desk at one of my surgeon's offices: If you wait more than 30 minutes to see your doctor, please inform the secretary. Your time is just as valuable as ours."

CHAPTER 25

"This Is Easy"

I'm 18 hours post-operative. This surgery was short, only two hours. We're all crossing our fingers that those marathon operations a couple months ago are over – for good.

But here I lay, hurting. Not from surgery, either. That'd be too easy. Now, I feel like my gut and bladder are ready to explode. I'm on plenty of narcotics to keep the surgical pain to a dull roar. Unfortunately, those narcotics have also shut down my ability to pee. Nurses and docs have told me before how anesthesia slows down bodily functions. Sometimes, I've heard, the body needs time to wake up... but narcotics keep my urinary track asleep. So, I can hurt like holy hell and pee, or I can be comfortable from surgical pain, but my bladder backs up. This is one of those damned if you do, damned if you don't scenarios.

"I just put in a call to Dr. Jones," the nurse says, crossing my room.

"He says if you're not able to urinate in an hour, we'll have to insert a foley."

Foley. I'm all too familiar with this trick. It's the ol' firehose up the pecker procedure. Getting a foley is traumatic for anyone. Double that trauma for a male. Triple it for a young guy who isn't used to exposing his junk to nurses. And quadruple the trauma when it's necessary to be done while the patient is awake. I've come out of surgery before with a foley hanging from my stuff, but this time it's going to be inserted while I'm awake – no good.

For an hour, I lay with a piss jug positioned between my thighs. I can't squeeze more than a couple drops. This will not do. The nurse enters again.

"Any luck?" she asks, sympathetically.

I shake my head furiously. I'm disgusted with this, but more than anything, I'm scared. The pressure in my bladder is so severe that I have to keep my head back, like the audience at an air show. It keeps my breathing passages more open and offers the tiniest bit of relief. I begin to feel sick… and that scares me even more. What if my bladder gets too stretched out? Could it rupture? If that would happen, would it mean more surgery? Would my insides be soaked in piss? Fear continues to creep up my neck as tears of discomfort and fear run down my cheeks.

"Okay, I'll get the foley, Marcus. I'll be right back." With that, she's gone. I'd run, if I could. But alas, I have a gut full of piss and a broken leg. I'm not running anywhere.

She returns and lays a couple of tubes across my legs.

"You're going to feel so much better in just a couple minutes, Marc," she says.

"I sure hope so," I gasp, internal pains stabbing at my stomach.

"Just to give you a little play by play here… I'm putting some KY on the end of the catheter so it'll be easier to insert. There's also some anesthetic on here to help with the discomfort," she says. Her words come quick, but she's working with her instruments all the while. I'm incredibly glad she can work and talk at the same time – especially when I'm hurting so much.

"I hate this," I cry, scared of getting this tube shoved where the sun don't shine. "Do you know what you're doing?" I'm pleading now.

"Absolutely, Marc. I know this is no fun, but this is one of the first things taught in nursing school. I'm really used to doing this, too. Foley catheters are so common after surgery and, well, this is a post-surgical floor. I do a couple of these every week. Now, are you ready?"

I nod. I just want her to get it over with. *Just do it*, I think. Nothing she can do, short of an amputation, can be worse than what I'm feeling now. I tilt my head back once again, take a couple steadying breaths and try to concentrate on something, anything, that is NOT happening in my lap.

⌒⌒

When performing a procedure on a patient, emphasize how easy the procedure is. Patients may take comfort in knowing the procedure is routine for the health care pro. Knowing it's not a complicated maneuver makes it easier to give up control. Keep the patient hopeful by reminding them how this procedure will help him/her feel better.

Plus, knowing the health care pro is experienced at said procedure just makes for a trifecta of comfort; it's easy, it'll help the patient feel better and it's something the health care pro does frequently.

CHAPTER 26

Fight Or Flight

"Come on, let's go, Marcus" the nurse says, hurrying me along.

I can barely move, much less move at a speed she wants me to go. I raise a palm in a "Slow down" posture and take a breath. I will not be rushed... but yet? She either doesn't get it or doesn't care.

"Come on, Marcus" she says, almost in a whine. Now, I'm angry. I gave her the opportunity to correct her prodding, but now she's just pissing me off.

"I'm going as fast as I can!" I bark at her.

"All right, all right," she says, sounding wounded that I'd taken a stronger tone with her. "You don't have to yell!" Now she is hurrying me AND scolding me. I am done being Mr. Nice guy.

"Dammit, I told you I'm going as fast as I can! Now get the hell off my back!"

Her hand, which had been around my bicep as she helped support me from the bed to the commode, tightens. Right or wrong, I take this as punishment; a spanking for being a bad boy. I steady myself with the opposite hand and yank my arm away from her. I throw a shoulder her way, hoping she'll back the hell off. She grabs at my arm again.

"Stop touching me!" I scream at her. It hurts to yell, but this isn't even close to what I want to do. A shoulder to the torso, an elbow cracking down onto her cheek bone and a hard right upper cut to her chin. I *want* to do this… and if I had better strength and balance, I might. As it is, I'm awkward and weak and unsteady. Screaming and yelling will have to suffice for physical blows. She takes a step back, reading my body language and finally – FINALLY listening to me. I regroup. I turn toward her.

"Don't you ever, EVER touch me again," I growl. "Do you understand me?" I begin to shake. Adrenaline pumps through my system. I am furious, nervous, excited and ready to kill.

At the writing of this chapter, I am 34 years old. It has been nearly a quarter century since I was in a fight. I don't enjoy violence, I've never been a fighter, hell, I probably wasn't a real great football player in high school because I didn't enjoy the idea of pummeling opposing players. Typically, I'm an even tempered guy who'd prefer to talk his way into agreements than argue out of one. And yet???

Patients are sorta like wounded animals. Actually, patients usually ARE wounded animals. They're totally out of their element, hurting, likely emotional, and they probably feel incredibly out of control and helpless. One of the first things one learns in psychology 101 is how nearly all creatures have the fight or flight mechanism.

Now, think of a typical patient… if they feel threatened, does fight or flight kick in? Absolutely… and due to being in an unfamiliar environment without their creature comforts, it probably kicks in earlier. But, can a patient take flight? With most hospitalized patients, no. They're likely recovering from surgery, or they're medicated, or infirm in some way. When fight or flight kicks in, and flight is not an option… what's left? You got it – fight.

We've all heard stories of health care professionals getting clocked or bitten, right? Kinda makes sense if the patient is on drugs or has been taken into protective custody for psychiatric reasons. But, there are plenty of examples of patients recovering from, say, a gall bladder procedure who have left nurses with a black eye. Why? They're helpless, out of control, scared and, yes, fight or flight kicked in. And with the inability to fly… that's what is left.

Simply be aware that flight is NOT an option for many patients. And when fighting persists, it's rooted in a feeling of severe vulnerability. If you can help the patient feel they retain some control, it eliminates a bit of that vulnerability. The less vulnerability, the less need for fight or flight. A bit of compassion, especially when a patient is helpless, goes a long, long way to protect their dignity… and your nose!

Chapter 27

"I'll Come Back Later"

A quiet hospital room, insomnia, a blind patient hurt too much to get out of bed. This is a great recipe for thinking. Or, maybe a bad idea to have so much time on my hands.

Tonight, I've listened to Bob Dylan while the hours ticked by. Every time I press the "talk" button on my new talking watch, another 30 minutes have passed. And I'm no closer to sleeping. I think and think and think. It's just me, Dylan, and my thoughts.

Even as much as I hurt, physically AND emotionally, I keep coming back to one conclusion: if there ever was a "good" time for something this horrible to happen, it's right now. Before the crash, I was physically stronger than I've ever been. That strength probably helped me survive. I have visual memory of my college campus. When I finally get back there, I'll be able to picture everything around me. I'm young and single – I'm not sure if I were married that any woman would have the strength to stick by my side. However, this time in my life is overflowing with friends. High school only ended six months ago, so I was still connected with my football buddies, fellow actors from the school play, members of my church youth group, etc. Plus, I had friends from camp, from college and, believe it or not, these nurses and docs are becoming my friends. Friends are simply everywhere.

Now, in this hospital room, I keep thinking over how much I appreciate all these friends. Finally, after hitting the talking watch a dozen times, I'm beginning to get sleepy.

Hours later, I wake to a familiar voice on my left.

"Engel, it's Woods. How ya doing, man?" John Woods, one of my friends since fourth grade. I nod, trying to wake up.

"I got some other guys along with me, dude," John says. One by one, five more high school buddies come up to my bed, state their name and shake my hand. I try to give a firm grip, a little sign to let them know I'm okay – I'm different, I'm changed, but I'm okay.

"What time is it?" I mumble.

"Just before noon," John says. "Hey, you mind if I throw on one of your CD's here?"

"Be my guest," I say, motioning towards the stereo. In moments, the licks of Jimmy Page's electric guitar begin to pour from the speakers.

"Zeppelin… always a good choice!" I say and hold my hand up for Woods to high five. The music loosens all of us up. Soon, it's like we're all just a bunch of guys hanging out. We can almost forget that one of us is blind and going through one of the most wretched human conditions imaginable… almost.

We talk and laugh. The guys have brought me some gifts: a U2 CD, a grip strength exerciser, a stuffed animal from one of their moms. I'm feeling really, really lucky.

There's a knock at the door. Barb steps in to see the crowd of guys and me laughing. She stops. I can almost hear the smile come over her face. "I'll come back later, Marc... you just keep having fun with your friends."

"Thanks, Barb," I call out over the music and give her a wave. She turns and walks out. Later, I learn that her exit was done with tears of joy in her eyes.

Everyone has a desire for human connection and relationships. Every single human, unless there's a screw loose up top, wants to feel supported, cared for and loved. This compassion and care is as valuable as whatever medicines the patient takes. Barb knew this. She also knew that whatever task she was to perform weren't nearly as important as a few good laughs with my buds.

If you have tasks that can wait, let your patient have their time with their loved ones. Laughter, conversation and that human connection can't be measured in milligrams or medical procedures, but in the comfort the patient derives from the love and support of those precious relationships.

CHAPTER 28

About Face

" I'm Dr. McAleer," a rushed voice said, swinging around the door into the exam room. His hurriedness frightens me. This wheelchair is none too sturdy and I don't have the strength to hold myself up if he comes crashing into me. Dr. McAleer plops down on his exam stool and opens my file. The file is on the desk, the desk faces a wall, the surgeon faces the wall.

This doc, an orthopedic surgeon or something, I don't know, has still never stopped by my room to introduce himself. Three surgeries, three different times I've laid on the OR table and he's operated. And three times he's never bothered to show up before the surgery to discuss what he'll be doing. I don't have a real favorable opinion of Dr. McAleer, anyway, but with no handshake and refusing to look at me, his approval rating is starting to go into negative integers.

"Dr. Braxton did the operation to put your legs in traction. I took them out of traction and attached the external fixator," he says, reading quickly over his notes in my file. It sounds like he's reminding himself to see what he's done and where he's been.

"Let's see... then I removed the external fixator, set the cast and inserted the IM nail. Does that all sound right?" he asks, scrawling a note on his paperwork.

"Well, I know that work was done..." I say. My implication is that, yes, I've been told that. But does a doctor need to be asking me, the patient, what he's done? My body is not your diary, doc.

"Are you still doing physical therapy?" he asks, disregarding my last answer.

"Yes," I say, gritting my remaining teeth. He makes another note.

"The X-rays show everything is fine from the IM nail. Do you have full range of motion back yet?" He is still scribbling notes, still hasn't looked up once.

"Almost. Every day it's getting a little better."

"Good. Keep doing the physical therapy. Your leg is now as good as new, maybe better than new with the artificial reinforcement of the IM nail. You can place as much weight on it as you can tolerate. Within a month, you should be able to walk with a support cane. When you're ready, you can stop using the walker. I'd like to see you back in six months." He makes one final notation, stands up, says, "Take care" and walks out the door. The encounter lasted less than three minutes. Not once did Dr. McAleer look at me.

Are you as troubled by this encounter as I was? To not even give a patient the simple courtesy and respect of looking him/ her in the eye is just pathetic. Was the doctor uncomfortable with my blindness? Did he not know how to react to looking at someone who could not look back at him? Maybe, but I doubt it. This simply felt like the doctor's usual method of patient care. Get in and get out. While an IM nail may be a common procedure for him, it is not for me, the patient.

No matter what is commonplace to a health care professional, unless the patient also works in that field, they want to know what's up. They want some interaction with their doctor. They want to know things the doctor knows, but what the doc may not be telling. Above all, they want to be treated like a person, not a procedure.

Think of it this way... would that doctor refuse to look the waitress at the coffeeshop in the face? His nurses? His wife? His colleagues? If so, a patient should know up front that this doctor has a "thing" about not looking people in the face. If not, never underestimate just what a negative message a refusal to face them sends to the patient.

CHAPTER 29

Shake A Hand, Shake A Hand

This is getting old. Another day, another journey to a new doctor's office. Never outside, never where I can feel and taste fresh air, never where I can get any sensation other than the pain and discomfort of being wheeled through this massive fortress of a hospital.

The orderlies arrive. The one near my head does the countdown, "One, two, three." On three, they hoist my sheet, my body, my being into the air like a drunkard asleep in a hammock. The sling squeezes my shoulders in and I hear the familiar crack of my ribcage. Strangely, it doesn't hurt. It's just disconcerting to hear my ribs cracking inside my chest.

Into the wheelchair, arrange the tubes, out into the hallway. Down the elevator, past the throngs of people rushing – always rushing – to be somewhere else.

We arrive at the doctor's office. The secretary says it should only be a few minutes. There are just a couple other patients in the waiting room. Either this doctor is such a specialist there are few patients, or he's not popular with patients. Or maybe there's another possibility. I try to give the doctor the benefit of the doubt, but I've been burned by so many other docs that I'm ready to throw the baby out with the bathwater.

True to her word, the secretary calls my name after just a few minutes. My parents help wheel me down the hallway to the examination room. The office nurse shows my parents where to place the wheelchair with me in it. Then she leaves saying, "The doctor will be in soon."

I have no idea what I'm doing here. *We already know I'm blind. What's the point of coming to another eye doctor? This doctor – some super duper specialist that Dr. Jones recommended, isn't going to be able to bring my sight back. No one can do that. Not the ophthalmologists, not me, not anyone. I'm simply blind. Forever. So why am I even here? This surgeon, Dr. Frey, what can he even do for me?*

I sit. I sit and I sulk. I try to take deep breaths to relax. I try to give this doctor the benefit of the doubt. I don't want to explode on him immediately like I've done with other doctors. Yet, I still cannot figure out what purpose it serves for me to go through all the discomfort of the transfer and be sitting here now.

There is a sound at the door. I hear the clipboard with my chart being lifted out of its plastic holder on the door. A second later the door opens.

"I'm Dr. Frey," a man's voice says. I extend my hand. He walks past me. My hand hangs in mid-air.

Is he still coming? I think. He steps past my parents, pulls out his rolling stool and sits down at the exam room desk. My hand is still there; still extended, still waiting for him to shake it.

The chart rattles onto the desk. I hear his pen scratching on paper. He's by-passed my handshake altogether. *Asshole,* I think. I let my hand drop to my lap.

"Dr. Jones recommended you see me?" he asks, pen still scratching on my chart. I nod. "Yes," my parents answer in unison.

More scratches of the pen. His back is to my parents. Since he's entered the room, he's never once glanced at them. Hell, he hasn't glanced at me.

"And your eyes were damaged in a motor vehicle accident?" he asks. The question is directed at me. Again I nod. The pen stops writing. He finally looks at me. I nod again. My parents jump in to answer his question. "Yes, several weeks ago." My dad blurts out. His attention is back on his paperwork. I slump in my chair. Less than 30 seconds into this encounter, I already hate this man.

In western culture, we are accustomed to two things when we are first introduced: shaking hands and exchanging names. Yet, why is the handshake not as prominently used in a health care setting as it is at, say a cocktail party?

Physicians take note: your levels of education, wealth and prestige are, at least, respected by your patients. At worst, they are intimidating. If a patient feels as though a physician refuses to shake his/her hand, the patient may perceive this as a personal insult.

In a hospital setting, a handshake gives most patients a feeling of normalcy. When a person is hospitalized, he/she does not feel anything close to normal. For most, the hospital is a new and different place. Obeying the common laws of courtesy go a very long way in increasing the comfort of your patients.

CHAPTER 30

Keep Your Promises

There's a knock at the door. My buddies, this time Jeff, David and Rodney, all turn to see who knocked. I turn, too, though my eyes see nothing – and never will again.

"Hi guys," says a cheery female voice. "Hi, Marcus. It's Jamie from physical therapy."

"Hey," I say, still smiling from whatever guy banter was flying before Jamie knocked.

"I see you've got your friends here now. I'll come back later and we can do your P.T."

"Sounds good," I say, turning back to face the guys. Jamie exits.

We talk. After another hour, we say our good-byes and they promise they'll be back next weekend. It's a two hour drive from the University of Missouri to Barnes Hospital – not exactly running out to the store for milk.

The guys leave. I wait for Jamie. An hour passes. No Jamie. Lunch arrives. I sift through the cream of wheat and tapioca pudding, some of the only things I can eat. The dietary staff returns to retrieve my lunch tray. No Jamie. Nurses take my vitals, change my dressings, help me give myself a sponge bath. Still no Jamie.

My parents arrive. Doctors make their evening rounds. I'm fine, everything is fine. More visitors arrive. Still no Jamie. Dinner arrives. Mashed potatoes and scrambled eggs and cream of broccoli soup. I eat the soup, injecting it into my mouth with a large plastic syringe. Dietary returns, retrieves the tray. Nurses change shifts. It's evening now and Barb is working tonight. I'm relieved and happy. Today has been a good day. But, I'm still waiting for Jamie.

I don't like P.T. It hurts and I feel unstable, like I could tumble over at any moment. Yesterday, for the first time, I'd maneuvered out of bed, across the room, into the hallway and down to the next room. When my hand finally touched the door frame, a sheen of sweat covered my forehead. I was elated! *Next time,* I'd said to myself, *I'm going to get to the next room down the hall – the other way.* Slowly but surely, day by day, I'd expand my world further and further. That had been my plan yesterday, at least.

Barb enters my room.

"Hey, buddy, how was your day?"

"Pretty good. Had some friends here and the docs said I'm doing good. Only thing is that Jamie from P.T. said she'd come back later. That was this morning. Any idea when she'll get here?"

"She said she'd be back later?" Barb inquires. I nod.

"Huh. That's kind of typical for P.T. They only work the day shift and they're on a pretty tight schedule. It's after seven, so I'm sure they're already gone for the day."

I sit, stunned. *No P.T.? But, how will I get better if the therapist won't even come back to work with me?*

111

"But...she...", I stammer, "She promised she'd come back later."

"I'm sorry, Marc. I know you're disappointed. I'll make a call to P.T., but I've never seen a physical therapist on the floor after five o'clock."

I sag into bed, disappointed, angry, sad.

In all actuality, Barb didn't even know Jamie. Jamie was a P.T., Barb was a nurse. Jamie worked days, Barb was strictly on night shift. But, Barb knew things I didn't; that the P.T'.s only worked a normal businessman's hours.

When I learned that Jamie would not be back, I was crushed. I'd had a banner day. I'd proven to myself, my family, my nurses and Jamie herself that I was getting stronger, day by day. While I had the momentum and motivation, I wanted to continue to work on P.T. I didn't want to risk regressing back to that battered hunk of human flesh unable to move in his hospital bed. Jamie held the key... and yet, her absence wouldn't let me unlock the door.

I was thankful Jamie had given me time with my friends, no doubt. However, rather than making a promise she could not fulfill, Jamie could have given me options.

"Marcus, I'm on a tight schedule today. I know you want time with your friends, so we can do a quick session of P.T. now... Or I can put you on the schedule first thing tomorrow morning." Any of the above options would have empowered me to further take control of my own therapy. Instead, Jamie had

failed to keep her promise. If she came back tomorrow, would I have the same motivation? Doubtful. Would I work as hard for her at P.T. as I would have today? Also doubtful. If another therapist came to work with me, would I give him/her 110% like I'd done with Jamie? Very unlikely.

If you tell a patient you'll do something, keep your word. Even something as small as a 30 minute P.T. session or getting the patient a carton of juice – if you say you'll do it, do your best to keep your promise.

CHAPTER 31

"Let's Work Together"

Today will be a completely new experience. A new doctor to examine my mouth. His name is Dr. Beehner.

I'm wheeled, less painfully this time, to his office and immediately ushered into an examination room. Nice, I think, as the orderly sets the brakes on my wheelchair. That's one good thing about this doc already – I don't have to wait.

A few minutes later, Dr. Beehner knocks on the door, enters, introduces himself, shakes hands all around and pulls up a stool next to me. His questions are all directed toward me. Even though I slur my words and speak as little as possible, it seems Dr. Beehner understands every word that comes from my lifeless lips. *Well, that makes sense, I think… he IS an oral surgeon. He probably sees tons of people who can't speak properly.*

Dr. Beehner looks into my oral cavity, asks plenty of questions about the freshly covered area along the roof of my mouth. He moves quickly, but carefully, gathering tons of information from questions as we go.

"Marcus, I think you're ready to have your jaws un-wired," he says, setting back to face me for a conversation.

"I am?" I slur, surprised.

"Yes, you are. I'm going to get a device to unhinge the hardware. Be right back," Dr. Beehner says, exiting the room and closing the door behind him.

"What do you think about that, Brother?" my dad asks excitedly. Using my childhood nickname, "Brother" is always a comfort, coming from him.

"I guess it's good," I say, anticipating how much this process is going to hurt.

Dr. Beehner reappears after just a minute. It seems he's already been anticipating my question. He pulls up his stool next to me, again ready for conversation before action.

"How this works, Marcus, is pretty simple. I have a device here that will release the wires that hold your jaws immobile. It may be a little uncomfortable while I'm in there, but it shouldn't be painful. I'm not puncturing your skin or touching anything that should excite the nerves in your face. Are you ready?" I nod.

The procedure is over quickly. Painful? Not really, but the anticipation of pain is sometimes worse than the pain itself.

"How was that?" Dr. Beehner asks, his work complete.

"Not bad," I say, feeling the unique sensations of a mouth without as much hardware.

"Good!" Dr. Beehner says, genuinely pleased.

"Now, Marcus, this is where you and I will really start to work together. Scar tissue has built up while your jaws have been wired shut. That scar tissue is preventing your jaws from opening as wide as they should." He pauses, letting this information sink in.

"Our job now is to break down that scar tissue. We'll create a set of exercises to help your jaw achieve the mechanical movement of a typical jaw, okay?"

I nod. I bite down, trying to feel how much my jaw moves now that the wires have been cut – not much. Not much at all.

"How do I do this?" I ask, afraid of the answer.

"It's really pretty simple. Here, I'll show you," he says, handing me a metal rod with a couple thick Velcro straps.

"This is a perpetual motion machine. If you feel down here," he says, guiding my hands to something that looks like a hard plastic mouth guard like I wore in football, "This is the part that exercises your jaw."

Dr. Beehner flips a tiny switch on the metal rod. The mouthpiece slowly begins to open, wider and wider. There is a quiet whir as the mouthpiece reaches its widest, then begins to shrink back together.

Any idiot can see that the two pieces will be inserted into my mouth, then the perpetual motion machine will move my jaw, just like using the floor jacks at my high school job at the Texaco station.

After a few more explanations Dr. Beehner slips the straps around my chin and forehead. He shows me how to fit the pieces into my mouth. Suddenly, my jaw is moving like it hasn't in weeks. It's not comfortable. In fact, it hurts like hell. But, even after a few seconds, I can tell the machine is meeting its intended purpose.

"Marcus, I know this isn't the most comfortable thing in the world, but if you and I can work together, we can get your jaw back in shape – I promise!"

What is your wording when communicating with your patients? Do you inform the patient what he/she must do? Or, do you try to create an atmosphere of teamwork?

Dr. Beehner, in every one of his communications, used terms like "we," "our" and "us." I truly felt like I had more than just a doctor looking out for my welfare, but someone who wanted the same thing as I. And when I am on a team, and the others are doing their part, it inspires me to want to do my part.

No one likes to take orders. Patients may even be more sensitive to this than Joe Average person on the street. The more your words highlight the team approach, the more the patient will feel like he/she isn't being ordered, but taught how to best take care of him/herself.

The fastest way to help create the teamwork feel is to watch your pronouns. We, our, us; these include all members of the treatment team. Patients are more likely to respond positively to an atmosphere of collaboration with their health care providers.

CHAPTER 32

"How's This Working For You?"

Dr. Beehner pays a surprise visit to my room. It's only been a few days since he unwired my jaws, and the TMJ perpetual motion machine actually seems to be working. I hate it, but it IS working.

"Hi, Marcus," he says, striding up to my bed and shaking my hand. "How are you doing?"

"Okay, I guess. This thing sucks." I point at the apparatus enveloping my head.

"Why is that?" Dr. Beehner asks, sounding truly concerned.

"It just does. It hurts, I feel like I'm gagging, I can't talk for an hour per day – it just sucks." I could go on and on, but I like Dr. Beehner.

"Yeah, with the oral damage you've suffered, your mouth is going to be a good deal more sensitive than many of the patients who use this machine. I understand it's uncomfortable, but how's it working for you?"

I describe the progress I'm making, show him the movement of my jaw. Dr. Beehner is pleased. Before he leaves, he says, "Keep doing what you're doing, Marcus... you're really making headway!"

Dr. Beehner made me and my comfort the focus of the inter-action. "How is this working for you?" Key words: "for you."

Many other doctors would have asked me, "Are you doing what you should? Are you using this machine like I told you? Are you following my orders?" These sorts of questions put the focus on the machine, the procedure and the doctor's orders; NOT on the patient. Phrasing questions to gauge the benefit to the patient helps the patient feel as though they, not the machine/procedure/medication are important.

Patients may be reluctant to use medical devices. Wheelchairs and walkers and canes may not be difficult for the patient to use, but they may associate a stigma with having to use such devices. Same with medical devices like the TMJ machine, sleep apnea machine, syringes, commodes. By keeping the focus on how the patient feels he or she has (or has not) ben-efitted, you're helping the patient understand the true value of the therapy – and that's a huge step toward having a compli-ant patient!

CHAPTER 33

"How Do You Feel About It?"

I sit here in the dentist's office. The chair is a typical dentist's chair: long, contoured, comfortable. But, the doctor with his fingers in my mouth is no average cavity filler. He doesn't do crowns and cleanings or tartar removal. He does, in fact, make things out of nothing. My mouth is nothing. Less than nothing.

My mouth is a pulverized mess of broken teeth fragments, nerve damage, exposed bone, blood and spit. The usual functions of a mouth are impossible; eating, speaking clearly, etc. Dr. Gay's job is to fix all that.

Dr. Gay is not just a dentist, but a *maxial facial prosthetic specialist*. He takes the mouths of people like me and gives them the ability to eat. We all need to eat, to talk, to smile, to kiss. Dr. Gay has been working with my mouth for months. The going is slow. I want it to be over... and it's close. Very close.

It started with simple examinations. Dr. Gay looked in my mouth, tried to pry my jaws open wider. They wouldn't budge. The pain was enormous. I screamed. I screamed and I cursed and insulted him. This man who was trying to help me got an earful of some of the most profane names a person can be called. He'd jerked me around like a rag doll. He'd forced my body to do things it couldn't. He'd shoved pointed, prying metal rods into my sensitive mouth. After the tirade, I didn't even know if he would see me again. And, if he weren't a last result, I wouldn't have ever stepped foot in his office again.

The next appointment, I didn't speak. Even when he asked me a direct question, I wouldn't respond. This, I thought, was an improvement from swearing at him. It was also an effort. I wasn't going to be the one to extend the olive branch, but I'd concede to being near when it was cut from the tree.

Months went by and things improved. I grew to respect Dr. Gay's talent. He grew to respect my dignity as a person, not just a patient.

Now, here we are… close to the end of the road. A new upper plate rests in my mouth. To fashion this plate, Dr. Gay was forced to do some of the most meticulous adjustments of his career. Limited jaw movement, loss of many teeth, osteo-integrated dental implants, crowning a cracked molar… and then, getting everything to work together properly.

The new upper plate has now been in my possession for two weeks. Before that, everything had to be pureed through a food processor. Now? I can eat solid food once again. I won't be chowing into a fat cheeseburger any time soon, but at least I can eat some foods. Not a lot, but more. Pasta, soft bread, french fries.

Here in Dr. Gay's office, it's time to check on my progress. A list of foods that are simple to eat, a list of things I can struggle through, a list of things that are still an impossibility.

Dr. Gay enters the room. He shakes my hand. His smile and greeting are warm, genuine. He pulls a rolling stool near my chair, not grabbing at any instruments or telling me to open my mouth. First, conversation.

"Well, Marcus, we're in the home stretch now. Last time you were here, we did some adjustments to the denture. I've looked over your lists of food and I'm glad you're able to start eating some regular food again." I nod.

"Aesthetically your mouth looks great! Your lips look full, you don't have the visual of a mouth being caved in. Anyone who isn't a dentist would never give it a second glance. So, I think we've accomplished one goal; aesthetic improvement. But the big question is this, Marcus: How do you feel about it?"

"Um, okay, I think. I'm glad I don't look like I have a fish mouth any more. Some things are hard to eat, but that might be jaw movement and nerve damage, too. It's kinda hard to tell which is the biggest problem."

"You're right, Marcus. There are so many pieces of this puzzle that is your mouth. This is why I'm here to do everything I can to be sure your mouth is as functional as possible. The more information you can give me, the more I can help you. So, I just need you to really explain to me how you feel about it, okay?"

⌒

Dr. Gay had two goals when working with my mouth: function and aesthetics. Functionally, every tiniest fraction of a milli-

meter had been accounted for. The adjustments of grinding parts, roughing other parts and keeping it all where pressure sores didn't form seemed a lot of plates to keep spinning.

Aesthetically, he AND my family were pleased with the results. One goal absolutely accomplished, second goal on the way. But, beyond the two goals of Dr. Gay appeared the best improvement of all: the doctor/patient relationship. His question, "How do you feel about it, Marcus?" put me back in the driver's seat. It was my mouth, my plate, my crown, my natural teeth and my ability to speak and eat.

Often times, doctors and nurses and therapists will work toward a certain goal or goals. Accomplishing that task becomes of paramount importance. Dr. Gay had his goals, too, but he would stop along the way to ask my opinion, "What do you think of this?"

Yes, my comfort was important, but his questions were for my morale as much as comfort. He allowed me to give my input, listened and adjusted his masterpiece as necessary. This question allowed me to take part in my own care and, hopefully, gave Dr. Gay extra information from the patient's perspective, not just footprints on the way to the summit of the mountain.

CHAPTER 34

"I Know What It Is, But Tell Me Anyway"

"Just going to slip this cuff over your arm and get your blood pressure, Marcus," says the nurse in Dr. Jones exam room.

"Okay," I say, raising my wrist to give her access.

The cuff tightens, then releases. She replaces it to its holder on the wall.

"Now, I'm just going to take a listen to your heart. Lean forward a little for me and you'll feel the stethoscope against your back – it might be kinda cold."

She's right – it is. I chuckle a little. As if anything can even be considered uncomfortable after the pain of the last couple months.

"Your vitals are all perfect. One last listen and I'll send in Dr. Jones," she says, scribbling on my chart.

"I'll need you to lay down all the way back. Here, I'll extend the table for your legs," she says. A cushioned pad is pulled out with a loud, metallic clunk. I ease down, my chest still feeling odd from the removal of ribs.

"I'm going to listen to your stomach and intestines. The stethoscope might still be a little cold, okay?"

I nod as the chilly circle lightly pushes into my abdomen.

"I don't get the chance to do this very often, Marcus," she says brightly.

"Get to?" I ask, a little confused.

"Yeah, get to. Most of Dr. Jones' patients have to be cleared for plastic surgery, so we know their vitals are healthy for the long term. Since you still have the feeding tube in, and since you had the swelling of your aorta, Dr. Jones has asked me to keep an extra eye on your vitals. When I was a floor nurse, I got to do it all the time, but now, I mainly assist Dr. Jones in the OR. It's kinda fun to take vitals again!"

Chit chat is a health care professional's best friend, as far as the patient is concerned. Interactions with patients can go much more smoothly the more the health care pro speaks to them, asks questions and informs them of what they're doing.

Practically any patient who has received treatment in the last 40 years would be able to visually spot a blood pressure cuff. Same story with a stethoscope. Same with a thermometer, though thermometer technology seems to change every week. When I was a kid, a thermometer was a single glass tube with a metal bulb. But think of all the other types of thermometers; the electronic thermometer with a cord to a power pack, the digital ear thermometer and, lately, a simple tool swiped across a patient's forehead. By the time you read this book, there may be something even more advanced!

Now, let's say you're a patient who hasn't been in the hospital in years. Maybe you haven't even been to the doctor in years.

Before you see the doctor, a nurse is standing at your side, shoving something into your ear. You have no idea what this is. Your only point of reference for a thermometer has been the old glass stick under the tongue. If the health care professional does NOT inform the patient what they are measuring, a golden opportunity is missed.

All in all, even if a patient knows what a certain instrument is for, tell them what you're doing, anyway. Tell them what information you're obtaining from their body. This information may help the patient relax and be more comfortable with the impending physician's visit. It may help them understand that the info you're gathering is something you do for every patient. It may give them comfort to know you take vitals 20 times per day. It may help the patient to know exactly what that blood pressure cuff is used for, even if they're in the office or hospital regularly.

Simply put, even if your patient is a regular, the office, the hospital, the treatment facility is still probably not in their comfort zone. The more info you can give the patient, the more comfortable they will be.

EPILOGUE

If you've read this far, there's a good chance you also read my first health care book, *The Other End Of The Stethoscope: 33 Insights For Excellent Patient Care.* If so, thank you! And if you've read my autobiography, *After This...,* thank you, too.

Nothing makes me happier than hearing feedback from my readers. I take comfort in the knowledge that others are reading these tips, learning from them and (hopefully) implementing them in their care of patients. If you've been able to take anything positive from what you've read here, then it was worth all the work, tedium and frustration that go with writing a book.

It's a joy, don't get me wrong, but it's a huge undertaking, too. What keeps me writing (and wanting to write) is the knowledge that my work is making a difference in the lives of patients. And maybe in the lives of health care professionals, too.

So, I'd REALLY love to hear from you if you've taken one of these insights to heart and implemented it into your healthcare practice. Drop me an e-mail at Marcus@ MarcusEngel.com, or look me up on FaceBook (www. Facebook.MarcusEngel.com) and let me know!

And as always, thank you. If you're in one of the roles that helped save my life, thank you. If you've committed your life to helping others, thank you. And if you've taken the time to read these words to help the patients under your care, thank you, too.

MPE

Marcus Engel is a professional speaker and bestselling author whose messages inspire, and honor health care professionals with insight and strategies for excellent patient care.

Marcus' memoir, *"After This...An Inspirational Journey for All the Wrong Reasons,"* chronicles his amazing life story and is the basis for *"The Drop,"* a multi-award winning short film that is currently in development as a feature film.

Marcus holds a B.S. in Sociology from Missouri State University and an M.S. in Narrative Medicine from Columbia University in the city of New York. He lives in Orlando, Florida with his wife, Marvelyne and Seeing Eye dog, Garrett. He is an avid reader, writer, musician and traveler, both on a professional level and just when he needs to get away.

For info on keynote speeches, Narrative Medicine Workshops, books, DVDs or just to say hi, please visit:
www.MarcusEngel.com

Take the pledge!

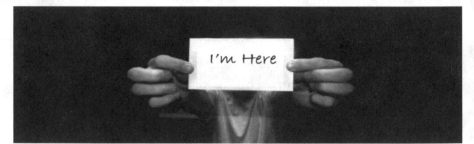

www.*ImHereMovement*.org

GET MARCUS' FREE MONTHLY NEWSLETTER RIGHT IN YOUR INBOX!
It's packed with information, inspiration,the latest "Marcus News" and fun contests to win cool prizes & one of a kind "Marcus Swag!"
Sign up at

www.MarcusEngel.com or just text the word "MARCUS" to 22828
And of course – we never ever spam or share your email address – EVER!

Marcus loves to interact with readers and is, in his own words, "a social media junkie."
Connect with him via:
Marcus@MarcusEngel.com
Twitter.com/MarcusEngel
FaceBook.com/MarcusEngelSpeaker